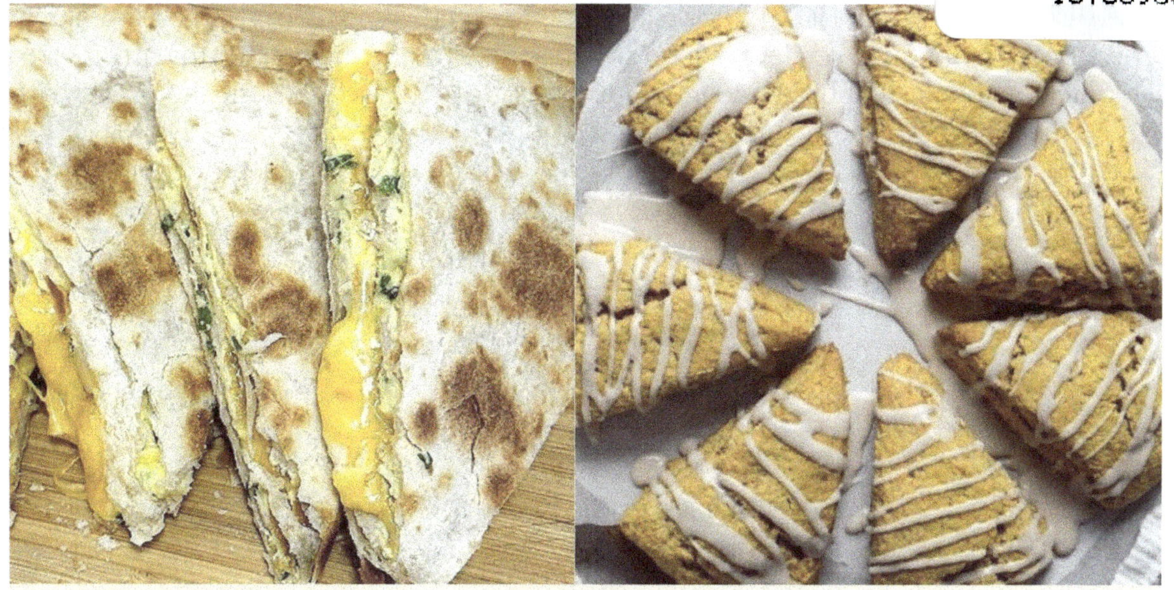

Gestational Diabetes
Cookbook

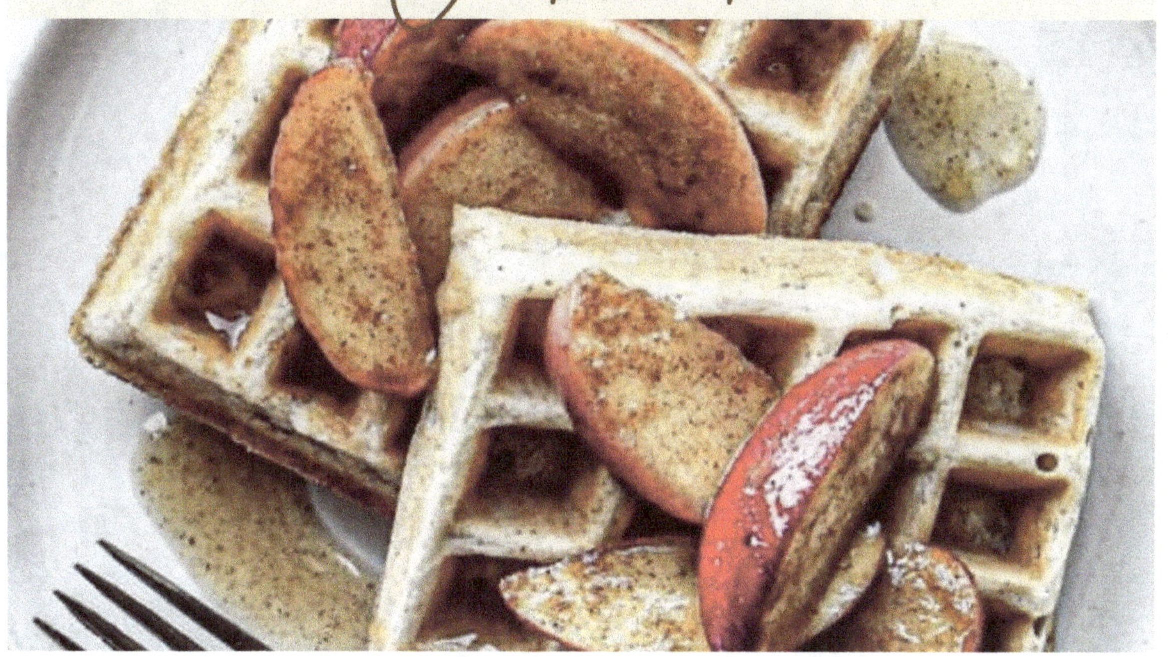

TABLE OF CONTENT

CHAPTER ONE: INTRODUCTION

What Is Gestational Diabetes?

GDM is a prevalent diagnosis among expectant mothers. According to the Centres for Disease Control and Prevention (CDC), 9.2% of pregnant women globally have GDM, and the number is rising. In addition to all of the excitement and anxieties that accompany pregnancy, receiving a diagnosis like GDM can be debilitating. It's critical to realize that your dietary choices most likely did not cause this disease. Although lean or obese women can develop gestational diabetes, being overweight is unquestionably associated with an increased risk of the disease. A diagnosis of gestational diabetes mellitus does not imply that you had diabetes before becoming pregnant or that you will always have this illness. Pregnancy-related GDM diagnosis may disappear after childbirth. When blood sugar, commonly known as blood glucose, is increased, GDM is diagnosed. Even though the precise etiology of GDM is uncertain, decreased insulin sensitivity is a known contributing factor. The placenta's hormones, which aid in the baby's development, also prevent the mother's insulin from functioning correctly. Put differently, the hormones that the placenta produces oppose the effects of insulin. To lower blood sugar levels, the pancreas secretes the hormone insulin, which transports glucose from the blood into your cells. Blood sugar levels stay high when insulin is unable to carry out its function as intended. Insulin resistance, also known as impaired insulin sensitivity, is a disease that often starts in the middle of pregnancy and gets worse as the pregnancy goes on. For this reason, the glucose tolerance test—a routine examination used by medical experts to diagnose GDM—is typically deferred until weeks 26 through 28 of pregnancy. (We'll talk about the test's protocol soon.) Usually, insulin resistance goes away right after having delivery.

Symptoms of GDM

Because the symptoms of GDM are so similar to those of pregnancy, people rarely recognise them. The three most prevalent symptoms are increased thirst, excessive urination, and fatigue.

Women may not be aware they have gestational diabetes mellitus (GDM) because the symptoms are usually undetectable or mistaken for typical pregnant symptoms. Usually, a standard glucose screening test is required to diagnose women with gestational diabetes.

Test for Glucose Tolerance

Usually conducted between weeks 26 and 28, the regular glucose screening test is also known as an oral glucose tolerance test or a sugar test. Your doctor or midwife may test you earlier if, during typical prenatal appointments, you have elevated glucose levels in your urine.

Causes of GDM

The exact cause of gestational diabetes in some women and not in others is still unknown to researchers. Overweight prior to conception frequently contributes. Normally, a number of hormones regulate blood sugar levels. However, hormonal changes that occur during pregnancy make it more difficult for the body to properly process blood sugar. This causes blood sugar levels to rise.

Gestational diabetes is commonly associated with the following signs in pregnant women, in addition to a mother's age of over 25:

BMI, or body mass index BMI is a weight-to-height ratio calculation. Both women with normal BMIs and obese women are diagnosed with gestational diabetes; however, the pathophysiology is different in the two groups:

- BMI in the obese range (30 or above). There is a correlation between increasing insulin resistance and obesity both before and at week 28 of pregnancy. Insulin resistance is thought to be caused by adipose tissue, or stored fat tissue. If you were overweight before to becoming pregnant, you probably had insulin resistance, but if you didn't have regular blood work done, you might not have been aware of it. Insulin resistance increases throughout pregnancy.
- BMI being within the usual range (18.5 to 24.9). Despite having a normal BMI, some women are susceptible to developing insulin resistance during pregnancy. However, compared to obese women, thin women usually do not exhibit pre-pregnancy insulin resistance.

Ethnicity: Compared to non-Hispanic white women, women who identify as African American, Hispanic American, Native American, Pacific Islander, and South or East Asian have a higher prevalence of GDM.

Diabetes's past: The chance of developing GDM is increased by a family history of diabetes, such as having a family member with type 1 or type 2 diabetes. Moreover, prediabetes before becoming pregnant or gestational diabetes from previous pregnancies raise the risk of GDM. Slightly raised blood glucose levels are indicative of prediabetes, a disease that increases the risk of developing type 2 diabetes. When the hemoglobin A1C level is between 5.7 and 6.4%, prediabetes is identified.

Polycystic Ovarian Syndrome (PCOS): Insulin resistance is a component of the metabolic syndrome that coexists in 50% of women with PCOS. Women with PCOS are more prone to develop type 2 diabetes. Because of this, they are usually regarded as high risk during pregnancy and are thus advised to adhere to a strict diet and avoid gaining too much weight (M.-L. Pan et al.).

Absence of Physical Activity: Having previously given birth to a child who weighed more than nine pounds (4.1 kg)

Complications of GDM

It has previously been discovered that women with gestational diabetes are at risk for and may experience complications from stillbirths. Stillbirth rates are currently lower than in the past, most likely as a result of improved GDM monitoring and treatment. I'll go over potential pregnancy, delivery, and postpartum issues on the pages that follow.

Disorders of Hypertension: Hypertensive conditions can develop in expectant mothers. They are more likely to develop in women with GDM. Preeclampsia, eclampsia, and gestational hypertension are the three stages of hypertensive diseases, ranging in severity from moderate to severe.

- **Gestational hypertension:** When a woman who had normal blood pressure before becoming pregnant experiences high blood pressure when she is more than 20 weeks along, it is known as gestational hypertension. Usually, 12 weeks after giving birth, blood pressure returns to normal. Similar to GDM, gestational hypertension typically has no accompanying symptoms, making it challenging to diagnose. Usually, the mildly elevated blood pressure has no negative effects on the mother or infant.

However, difficulties might arise when gestational hypertension advances to preeclampsia, which affects 15 to 25% of women (P. Saudan, et al.).

- **Preeclampsia**, often called toxemia, may arise in the latter part of pregnancy, marked by elevated blood pressure reaching or surpassing 140/90 mmHg, heightened swelling, an excess of protein in urine, and abnormal placental development. It poses potential threats to both mother and baby, and the only remedy is delivering the baby. Some doctors recommend giving birth at 37 weeks, but unforeseen preterm labor before that threshold can also occur.
- **Eclampsia**, a severe escalation of blood pressure impacting the mother's brain function, can lead to seizures or even a coma. Preeclampsia or eclampsia may result in damage to the liver and blood cells, manifesting as HELLP syndrome. HELLP comprises Hemolysis, where oxygen-carrying red blood cells break down; Elevated Liver enzymes indicating liver damage, and Low Platelet count, signifying a reduced number of platelets, essential for preventing bleeding.

Complications during Delivery

Gestational diabetes may heighten the likelihood of a cesarean section (C-section) due to fetal macrosomia, referring to newborns with birth weights exceeding 8 pounds and 13 ounces, irrespective of gestational age. The surplus body fat is linked directly to the excess sugar in the mother's body, as the baby absorbs sugar beyond the body's metabolic capacity. A study revealed a clear connection between gestational diabetes and C-section rates: 19.5% of women with gestational diabetes underwent non-elective C-sections, compared to 13.5% for non-diabetic women (U. Kampmann, et al.).

Another potential complication is shoulder dystocia, occurring during delivery when the shoulders fail to follow the head in obstructed labor. There's a correlation between increased fetal size and the risk of shoulder dystocia.

Postpartum Type 2 Diabetes

Gestational diabetes can predispose you to postpartum disorders, increasing the risk of developing type 2 diabetes later in life. While blood sugars may normalize after delivery, the risk persists. Monitoring postpartum blood sugar levels through routine blood work and annual fasting glucose tests is crucial.

Type 2 diabetes, the most prevalent form, differs from type 1 and GDM. In type 1 diabetes, the body doesn't produce insulin due to an autoimmune attack on the pancreas's insulin-producing beta cells. Without insulin, blood sugar remains high. Type 1 diabetes management involves daily insulin injections or an insulin pump mimicking the pancreas's function by delivering small, continuous insulin doses under the skin throughout the day.

In type 2 diabetes, the body can produce insulin, but either insufficient amounts are made or the insulin is not used efficiently, leading to insulin resistance. Continuous exposure to sugar, common in the Standard American Diet (SAD), desensitizes cells to insulin's blood sugar-lowering effects. Imagine it as cells being bombarded with insulin, causing them to lose their ability to efficiently extract sugar from the blood, resulting in elevated blood sugar levels.

Type 2 diabetes is both preventable and reversible, with diet and lifestyle playing crucial roles. Balanced meals comprising unprocessed carbohydrates, protein, and healthy fats, along with limiting added sugar intake, can reduce the risk of developing type 2 diabetes. However, uncontrolled blood sugars may necessitate medication, and in severe cases, insulin therapy may be introduced.

Postpartum Cardiovascular Disease

Women with a history of gestational diabetes face a roughly 70% higher risk of cardiovascular disease (CVD), encompassing conditions like heart attacks, strokes, heart failure, abnormal heartbeat, and aortic stenosis. The development of type 2 diabetes, increased risk of metabolic syndrome, and vascular dysfunction contribute to the onset of CVD. Vascular dysfunction involves issues with large arteries (atherosclerosis), microcirculation, and endothelial dysfunction. Preventing type 2 diabetes is key to reducing the risk of CVD.

Healthy lifestyle changes post-pregnancy also play a crucial role: quitting smoking, moderating alcohol intake, maintaining a balanced diet with increased fruit and vegetable consumption, limiting processed foods, reducing excessive dining out, prioritizing physical activity, achieving a healthy weight, managing stress, and overall, taking care of mental and physical well-being. In essence, adopting a healthy lifestyle can prevent or slow the progression of nutrition-related diseases after pregnancy.

How GDM Affects Baby

Gestational diabetes (GDM) doesn't cause birth defects as it's diagnosed later in pregnancy, but poorly controlled GDM can impact the baby. High maternal blood glucose passes through the placenta, elevating the baby's blood glucose levels. The baby's pancreas produces extra insulin, storing excess energy as fat, potentially resulting in macrosomia (a large baby) and an increased likelihood of C-section.

Babies of mothers with GDM face higher risks of metabolic diseases in later life, including obesity, type 2 diabetes, and metabolic syndrome. Research suggests that high fetal insulin levels might influence the infant's growth and future metabolism. A U-shaped graph relating birth weight to the risk of type 2 diabetes indicates that both decreased and increased birth weights elevate the risk, while normal birth weight poses no risk.

GDM can also lead to newborns having very low blood glucose levels (hypoglycemia) at birth due to consistently high maternal blood glucose levels. This is because the fetus, accustomed to high insulin levels, continues producing it even when maternal glucose supply diminishes. Hypoglycemic newborns may receive glucose through an IV to raise blood levels. Additionally, excess insulin in the baby's body can hinder surfactant production, crucial for lung maturity, potentially causing breathing problems after birth.

Preventions

Preventing gestational diabetes isn't guaranteed, but adopting healthy habits before pregnancy can significantly help. If you've had gestational diabetes, these choices may also lower the risk of recurrence or developing type 2 diabetes in the future:

Eat healthy foods: Opt for high-fiber, low-fat, and low-calorie foods. Prioritize fruits, vegetables, and whole grains, ensuring variety without compromising taste or nutrition. Keep an eye on portion sizes.

Stay active: Exercise before and during pregnancy can reduce the risk of gestational diabetes. On most days of the week, aim for 30 minutes of moderate activity. Activities like brisk walks, cycling, or swimming, as well as short bursts like parking farther away, contribute to overall fitness.

Start pregnancy at a healthy weight: If planning pregnancy, shedding extra weight beforehand can promote a healthier pregnancy. Focus on lasting changes in eating habits, emphasizing more vegetables and fruits.

Control weight gain: While some weight gain in pregnancy is normal and healthy, gaining too much too quickly raises the risk of gestational diabetes. Consult your healthcare provider for personalized advice on reasonable weight gain for you.

Natural Treatments for GDM

Lifestyle changes form the foundation of natural treatment for gestational diabetes (GDM), often serving as the primary intervention before considering medication. This approach involves a blend of nutrition counseling and education, led by a registered dietitian or certified diabetes educator, along with physical activity and self-monitoring of blood glucose.

Self-monitoring entails frequent testing of blood sugar throughout the day, both before and after meals. This is done by drawing blood from your finger and placing it on a strip that displays the blood glucose level. Maintaining a blood sugar and diet log becomes crucial, aiding in identifying foods causing spikes and recognizing times when blood sugar tends to be elevated, such as in the morning. Armed with this information, you can better manage insulin dosage, if applicable, or choose foods that help maintain blood sugar within the appropriate range.

Vitamin D

There's a growing body of evidence suggesting a potential link between vitamin D deficiency and gestational diabetes (GDM), maternal obesity, and adverse outcomes for both mother and baby. The molecular and cellular mechanisms behind this association are only partially understood, and further research is needed to determine if vitamin D supplementation can reduce the risk of developing GDM or improve blood sugar control in affected women.

Regardless, maintaining optimal vitamin D levels is crucial. Prenatal supplements may not always provide sufficient vitamin D, which plays a role in supporting your immune function, healthy cell division, bone health, and aiding in the absorption of calcium and phosphorus. Additionally, for the baby, vitamin D is essential for promoting healthy bone development.

Calcium

Research indicates that higher dietary calcium intake, specifically from food (not supplements), is associated with a reduced risk of gestational diabetes (GDM). For women with a calcium intake below 1,200 milligrams per day, a daily increase of 200 milligrams was linked to a 22% reduction in GDM risk. This suggests a correlation between higher calcium intake and a lower risk of GDM.

Calcium is crucial during pregnancy as it not only helps reduce the risk of hypertension and preeclampsia but also supports various systems in the body, including musculo-skeletal, nervous, and circulatory systems. Your baby relies on calcium for building strong bones, teeth, nerves, muscles, and a healthy heart. Inadequate calcium intake may lead the baby to draw it from your bones, increasing the risk of developing osteoporosis later in life. Include calcium-rich foods like yogurt, cheese, sardines, kale, broccoli, bok choy, okra, and almonds in your diet, and consult your doctor about the need for calcium supplements.

Stress Management

Stress significantly impacts health and well-being, directly affecting hormone and blood sugar levels. It's essential to recognize the importance of managing stress for both you and your baby. Utilize tools like yoga, meditation, walking, journaling, self-care, or alone time to find what works best for you. Allocating as little as 20 minutes per day to stress reduction can make a significant difference during pregnancy, a potentially high-stress period. Acknowledge and prioritize managing stress, as it plays a crucial role in maintaining overall health and a positive pregnancy experience.

Nutrition Guidelines

Carb Counting

Carb counting, whether measured in grams or using carb counts, is a method to manage your blood sugar levels. Dietitians may suggest counting grams of carbs per meal or following portion guidelines, such as limiting carbohydrates to 1 cup per meal. The key is to choose the method that makes the most sense and is easiest for you to follow. Regardless of the approach, understanding proper portions and measuring your food aids in blood sugar control. Your meal plan may allow for a specific number of grams of carbs per meal, like 30 or 45 grams. Reading Nutrition Facts labels on packaged foods helps identify carb content, with 15 grams of carbs equaling 1 carb count. For foods without labels, like fruits and vegetables, measuring portions remains the best way to determine carbohydrate consumption.

Fiber

Focusing on fiber can help stabilize blood sugar levels. If a food contains more than 5 grams of dietary fiber, you can subtract half of the fiber grams from the total carbohydrate grams. For instance, with split peas:
- Carbohydrates: 19g
- Fiber: 7g

Subtracting half of the total fiber (3.5g) from 19g of carbs results in 15.5g of carbs. Referring to the chart, this falls into the category of 1 carb count. Embracing fiber-rich foods can be an effective strategy in managing blood sugar levels.

Meal Timing

Consuming several small meals and snacks throughout the day, totaling three meals and at least two snacks, is crucial for stabilizing blood glucose levels effectively. This approach supports better glucose control compared to larger, infrequent meals.

Consistency in meal timing is equally important, aligning with the body's natural daily rhythm. Organs like the stomach, intestines, pancreas, and liver operate optimally when synchronized, enhancing glucose control. A regular meal schedule prevents skipping meals, avoiding extreme hunger that might lead to consuming large, carb-heavy meals. This consistency promotes clearer thinking and facilitates healthier food choices, steering away from impulsive and less nutritious options that might occur when overly hungry. Maintaining a routine helps support stable blood sugar levels and overall well-being..

Testing Blood Sugars

Testing your blood sugar four times a day, before breakfast and two hours after each meal, is a common recommendation. Practitioners typically set blood sugar goals, such as 95 mg/dL or less before a meal (pre-prandial) and 120 mg/dL or less two hours after a meal (post-prandial).

Keeping a detailed log of your meals and corresponding blood sugar readings is essential. Your practitioner may provide a sample meal/blood sugar log to help you track and manage your levels effectively. Regular monitoring and documentation play a key role in maintaining control and ensuring your gestational diabetes management plan is on track.

Sample of blood sugar log

Date			
	Blood Sugar	Insulin Dose	Grams Carbs
Breakfast			
Snack			
Lunch			
Snack			
Dinner			
Snack			
Exercise			

Greek Yogurt Parfait

Prep Time: 10 minutes
Cook Time: 0 minutes
Total Time: 10 minutes
Servings: 2

Ingredients
- 1 cup Greek yogurt (low-fat)
- 1/2 cup fresh berries (blueberries, strawberries)
- 2 tablespoons chopped nuts (almonds, walnuts)
- 1 tablespoon chia seeds
- 1 teaspoon honey (optional)
- 1/2 teaspoon vanilla extract
- Dash of cinnamon

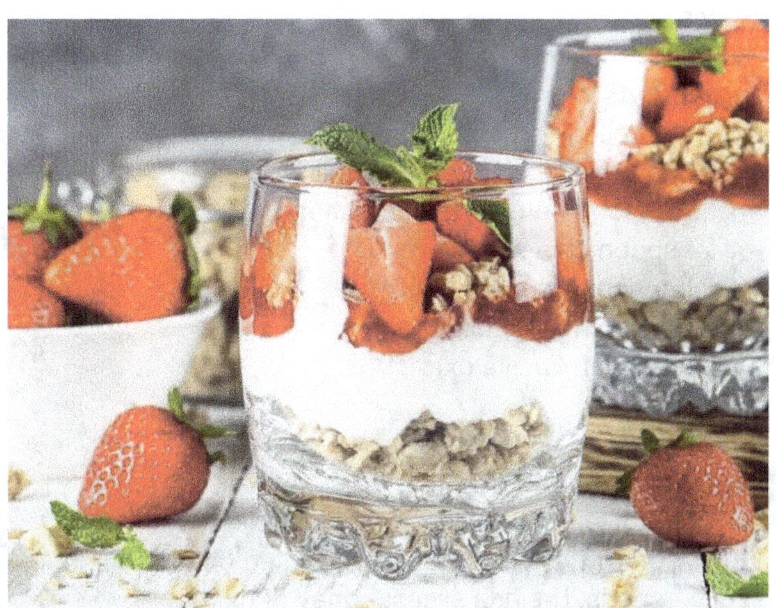

Instructions
1. In a bowl, mix Greek yogurt with vanilla extract until smooth.
2. In serving glasses or bowls, layer the Greek yogurt, fresh berries, chopped nuts, and chia seeds.
3. Repeat the layers until the glass is filled, ending with a dollop of Greek yogurt on top.
4. Drizzle honey on the surface for sweetness, if desired.
5. Sprinkle a dash of cinnamon for extra flavor.
6. Serve immediately and enjoy this delightful gestational diabetes-friendly treat!

Nutritional Values (per serving)
- Calories: 250 kcal
- Protein: 15g
- Carbohydrates: 20g
- Dietary Fiber: 5g
- Sugars: 12g
- Fat: 12g
- Saturated Fat: 2g
- Cholesterol: 10mg
- Sodium: 50mg

Peanut Butter Overnight Oats

Prep Time: 5 minutes
Cook Time: 0 minutes (overnight soaking)
Total Time: 8 hours (overnight soaking)
Servings: 1

Ingredients
- 1/2 cup rolled oats
- 1/2 cup unsweetened almond milk
- 1 tablespoon natural peanut butter
- 1 teaspoon chia seeds
- 1/2 banana, sliced
- 1 teaspoon honey (optional)
- 1/2 teaspoon vanilla extract
- Pinch of salt

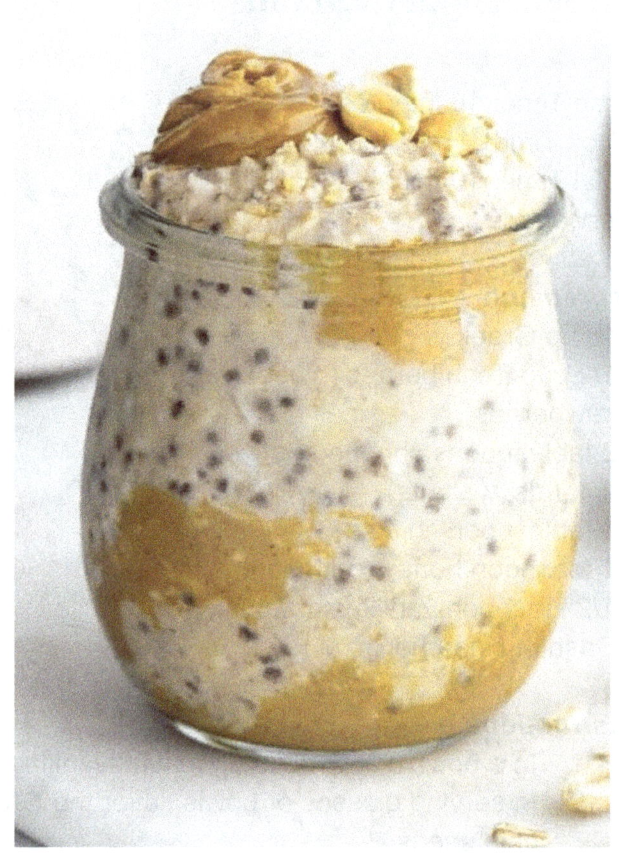

Instructions
1. In a jar or container, combine rolled oats, almond milk, peanut butter, chia seeds, banana slices, honey (if using), vanilla extract, and a pinch of salt.
2. Stir well to ensure all ingredients are evenly distributed.
3. Seal the jar or container and refrigerate overnight, allowing the oats to soak and flavors to meld.
4. In the morning, give the oats a good stir before serving.
5. Top with additional banana slices or a drizzle of peanut butter if desired.
6. Enjoy these delicious and gestational diabetes-friendly Peanut Butter Overnight Oats!

Nutritional Values (per serving)
- Calories: 350 kcal
- Protein: 12g
- Carbohydrates: 45g
- Dietary Fiber: 8g
- Sugars: 12g
- Fat: 15g
- Saturated Fat: 2g
- Cholesterol: 0mg
- Sodium: 180mg

High Protein Pancakes

Prep Time: 15 minutes
Cook Time: 10 minutes
Total Time: 25 minutes
Servings: 2

Ingredients
- 1 cup oat flour
- 1 scoop vanilla protein powder
- 1 teaspoon baking powder
- 1/2 teaspoon cinnamon
- 1/2 cup Greek yogurt (low-fat)
- 2 eggs
- 1 teaspoon vanilla extract
- 1-2 tablespoons almond milk (as needed for batter consistency)
- Cooking spray for pan

Instructions
1. In a bowl, whisk together oat flour, protein powder, baking powder, and cinnamon.
2. In a separate bowl, beat the eggs and then add Greek yogurt and vanilla extract. Mix until smooth.
3. Combine the wet and dry ingredients, adding almond milk gradually until you achieve a thick but pourable batter.
4. Heat a non-stick skillet or griddle over medium heat and lightly coat with cooking spray or oil.
5. Pour 1/4 cup portions of batter onto the skillet, spreading it out into a round shape.
6. Cook until bubbles form on the surface, then flip and cook the other side until golden brown.
7. Repeat with the remaining batter.
8. Serve the pancakes with your favorite berries or a dollop of Greek yogurt.

Nutritional Values (per serving)
- Calories: 320 kcal
- Protein: 25g
- Carbohydrates: 30g
- Dietary Fiber: 5g
- Sugars: 2g
- Fat: 12g
- Saturated Fat: 3g
- Cholesterol: 190mg
- Sodium: 300mg

Chia Seed Pudding with Raspberries

Prep Time: 5 minutes
Chill Time: 4 hours (or overnight)
Total Time: 4 hours and 5 minutes (or overnight)
Servings: 2

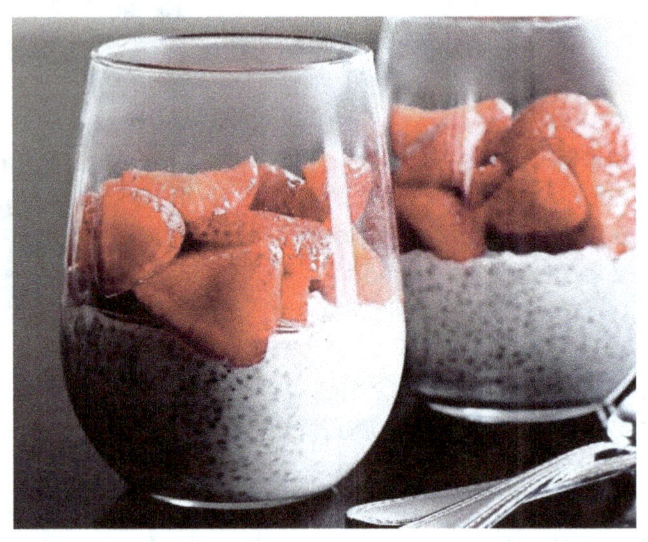

Ingredients
- 1/4 cup chia seeds
- 1 cup unsweetened almond milk
- 1 tablespoon maple syrup (optional)
- 1/2 teaspoon vanilla extract
- A pinch of salt
- 1/2 cup fresh raspberries
- Sliced almonds for garnish

Instructions
1. In a bowl, combine chia seeds, almond milk, maple syrup (if using), vanilla extract, and a pinch of salt.
2. Whisk the mixture thoroughly to avoid clumps and ensure even distribution of chia seeds.
3. Let the mixture sit for 5 minutes, whisking again to prevent clumping.
4. Cover the bowl and refrigerate for at least 4 hours or overnight, allowing the chia seeds to absorb the liquid and form a pudding-like consistency.
5. Stir the chia pudding well before serving.
6. Spoon the pudding into serving glasses or bowls.
7. Top with fresh raspberries and sliced almonds.
8. Drizzle a bit of additional maple syrup on top if desired.
9. Enjoy this delightful and nutrient-packed Chia Seed Pudding with Raspberries!

Nutritional Values (per serving)
- Calories: 180 kcal
- Protein: 5g
- Carbohydrates: 20g
- Dietary Fiber: 10g
- Sugars: 6g
- Fat: 9g
- Saturated Fat: 1g
- Sodium: 80mg

Breakfast Burritos

Prep Time: 15 minutes
Cook Time: 10 minutes
Total Time: 25 minutes
Servings: 2

Ingredients
- 4 large eggs, beaten
- 1 cup egg whites
- 1/2 cup diced bell peppers (any color)
- 1/2 cup diced tomatoes
- 1/4 cup diced onions
- 1/4 cup chopped spinach
- 1/2 cup black beans, drained and rinsed
- 1/2 teaspoon cumin
- Salt and pepper to taste
- 2 whole wheat or low-carb tortillas
- Salsa for serving (optional)
- Avocado slices for garnish (optional)

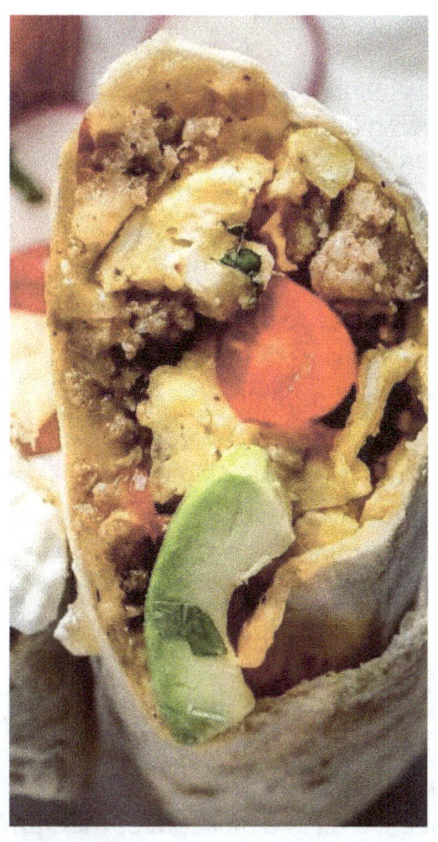

Instructions
1. In a skillet over medium heat, sauté diced onions until translucent.
2. Add bell peppers, tomatoes, and spinach to the skillet, cooking until vegetables are tender.
3. In a bowl, whisk together eggs, egg whites, cumin, salt, and pepper.
4. Pour the egg mixture over the vegetables in the skillet.
5. Stir gently until the eggs are cooked through and scrambled.
6. Add black beans to the skillet, stirring until heated.
7. Warm the tortillas in a dry pan or microwave.
8. Spoon the egg and vegetable mixture onto each tortilla.
9. Roll up the tortillas, creating breakfast burritos.
10. Serve with salsa and garnish with avocado slices if desired.

Nutritional Values (per serving)
- Calories: 380 kcal
- Protein: 30g
- Carbohydrates: 32g
- Dietary Fiber: 8g
- Sugars: 4g
- Fat: 14g
- Saturated Fat: 3g
- Sodium: 550mg

Tofu & Veggies Scramble

Prep Time: 10 minutes
Cook Time: 15 minutes
Total Time: 25 minutes
Servings: 2

Ingredients
- 1 block firm tofu, crumbled
- 1 tablespoon olive oil
- 1/2 cup diced bell peppers
- 1/2 cup cherry tomatoes, halved
- 1/4 cup diced red onions
- 1/2 cup chopped spinach
- 2 cloves garlic, minced
- 1/2 teaspoon turmeric (for color)
- Salt and pepper to taste
- Parsley or cilantro for garnish
- Whole grain toast or tortillas for serving

Instructions
1. Heat olive oil in a skillet over medium heat.
2. Add diced onions and minced garlic, sautéing until fragrant.
3. Add crumbled tofu to the skillet, sprinkling turmeric for color.
4. Cook tofu for 5-7 minutes, stirring occasionally.
5. Add diced bell peppers, cherry tomatoes, and chopped spinach to the skillet.
6. Cook for an additional 5-8 minutes, or until vegetables are tender.
7. Season with salt and pepper to taste.
8. Garnish with fresh herbs.
9. Serve the tofu and veggies scramble on whole grain toast or inside tortillas.

Nutritional Values (per serving)
- Calories: 280 kcal
- Protein: 20g
- Carbohydrates: 12g
- Dietary Fiber: 4g
- Sugars: 4g
- Fat: 18g
- Saturated Fat: 2g
- Cholesterol: 0mg
- Sodium: 300mg

Quinoa Porridge

Prep Time: 5 minutes
Cook Time: 15 minutes
Total Time: 20 minutes
Servings: 2

Ingredients
- 1/2 cup quinoa, rinsed
- 1 cup almond milk (unsweetened)
- 1/2 teaspoon cinnamon
- 1/4 teaspoon nutmeg
- 1 tablespoon maple syrup (optional)
- 1/4 cup chopped nuts (almonds, walnuts)
- 1/4 cup fresh berries (blueberries, strawberries)
- 1 tablespoon chia seeds
- Greek yogurt for topping (optional)

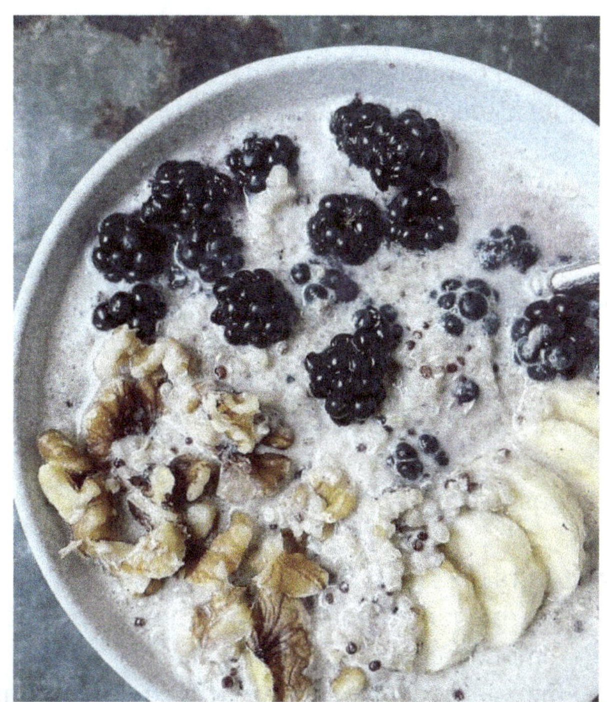

Instructions
1. In a saucepan, combine quinoa and almond milk.
2. Bring to a boil, then reduce heat to low, cover, and simmer for 15 minutes or until quinoa is cooked and most of the liquid is absorbed.
3. Stir in cinnamon, nutmeg, and maple syrup if desired.
4. Remove from heat and cover it for 5 mins
5. Fluff the quinoa with a fork and divide it between serving bowls.
6. Top with chopped nuts, fresh berries, and chia seeds.
7. Add a dollop of Greek yogurt if you like.
8. Drizzle with additional maple syrup for sweetness, if desired.

Nutritional Values (per serving)
- Calories: 320 kcal
- Protein: 10g
- Carbohydrates: 45g
- Dietary Fiber: 7g
- Sugars: 10g
- Fat: 12g
- Saturated Fat: 1g
- Cholesterol: 0mg
- Sodium: 150mg

Protein Smoothie

Prep Time: 5 minutes
Total Time: 5 minutes
Servings: 1

Ingredients
- 1 scoop vanilla protein powder
- 1 cup unsweetened almond milk
- 1/2 banana
- 1/2 cup frozen berries (blueberries, raspberries)
- 1 tablespoon almond butter
- 1/2 teaspoon chia seeds
- Ice cubes (optional)

Instructions
1. In a blender, combine vanilla protein powder, almond milk, banana, frozen berries, almond butter, and chia seeds.
2. If desired, add ice cubes for a colder and thicker consistency.
3. Blend until smooth and creamy.
4. Serve in a glass cup.

Nutritional Values (per serving)
- Calories: 350 kcal
- Protein: 25g
- Carbohydrates: 30g
- Dietary Fiber: 8g
- Sugars: 12g
- Fat: 15g
- Saturated Fat: 1g
- Cholesterol: 0mg
- Sodium: 250mg

Egg Muffins

Prep Time: 10 minutes
Cook Time: 15 minutes
Total Time: 25 minutes
Servings: 2 (6 muffins)

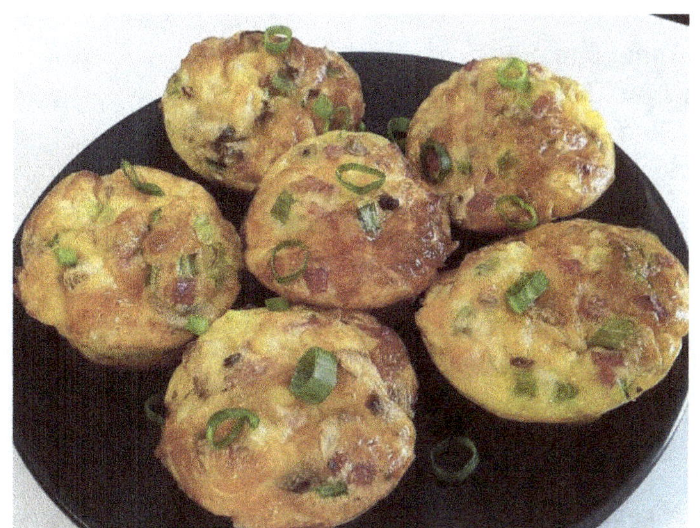

Ingredients
- 4 large eggs
- 1/4 cup milk (or almond milk)
- 1/2 cup diced bell peppers (color variety)
- 1/4 cup diced onions
- 1/4 cup chopped spinach
- 1/4 cup grated cheese (cheddar or feta)
- Salt and pepper to taste
- Olive oil or cooking spray

Instructions
1. Preheat the oven to 350°F (180°C).
2. In a bowl, whisk together eggs and milk until well combined.
3. Stir in diced bell peppers, onions, chopped spinach, and grated cheese.
4. Season with salt and pepper to taste.
5. Grease a muffin tin with cooking spray or olive oil.
6. Pour the egg mixture evenly into each muffin cup.
7. Bake for 15 minutes or until the eggs are set and lightly browned on top.
8. Allow the egg muffins to cool slightly before removing them from the muffin tin.
9. Serve warm and enjoy these delightful Egg Muffins!

Nutritional Values (per serving - 3 muffins)
- Calories: 250 kcal
- Protein: 18g
- Carbohydrates: 8g
- Dietary Fiber: 2g
- Sugars: 4g
- Fat: 15g
- Saturated Fat: 6g
- Cholesterol: 370mg
- Sodium: 450mg

Hard Boiled Eggs with Soldiers

Prep Time: 5 minutes
Cook Time: 8 minutes
Total Time: 13 minutes
Servings: 2

Ingredients
- 4 large eggs
- 4 slices whole grain bread, toasted and cut into strips (soldiers)
- Salt and pepper to taste

Instructions
1. Put the eggs in a saucepan covered with water
2. Bring water to a boil, then reduce heat to a simmer and cook eggs for 8 minutes.
3. Remove eggs from hot water and transfer them to a bowl of cold water to cool.
4. Once cooled, peel the eggs and cut them in half lengthwise.
5. Season the eggs with salt and pepper.
6. Serve the hard-boiled eggs with whole grain toast soldiers for dipping.

Nutritional Values (per serving)
- Calories: 250 kcal
- Protein: 15g
- Carbohydrates: 20g
- Dietary Fiber: 4g
- Sugars: 2g
- Fat: 12g
- Saturated Fat: 3g
- Cholesterol: 380mg
- Sodium: 450mg

Breakfast Tostada

Prep Time: 10 minutes
Cook Time: 10 minutes
Total Time: 20 minutes
Servings: 2

Ingredients
- 2 whole grain or corn tostadas
- 4 large eggs

- 1/2 cup black beans, drained and rinsed
- 1/2 avocado, sliced
- 1/4 cup diced tomatoes
- 1/4 cup diced onions
- 1/4 cup chopped cilantro
- 1 lime, cut into wedges
- Salsa for topping
- Salt and pepper to taste

Instructions
1. Heat the tostadas in a dry skillet or oven until crisp.
2. In a separate skillet, cook eggs to your liking (fried or scrambled).
3. Warm the black beans in the same skillet or microwave.
4. Place a tostada on each plate and top with black beans, eggs, avocado slices, diced tomatoes, onions, and cilantro.
5. Season with salt and pepper.
6. Serve with lime wedges and salsa on the side.

Nutritional Values (per serving)
- Calories: 400 kcal
- Protein: 18g
- Carbohydrates: 35g
- Dietary Fiber: 12g
- Sugars: 4g
- Fat: 22g
- Saturated Fat: 4g
- Cholesterol: 370mg
- Sodium: 480mg

Callaloo Frittata

Prep Time: 15 minutes
Cook Time: 20 minutes
Total Time: 35 minutes
Servings: 4

Ingredients
- 6 large eggs
- 1 cup callaloo (amaranth or spinach can be a substitute), chopped
- 1/2 cup diced bell peppers (any color)
- 1/4 cup diced onions
- 1/4 cup diced tomatoes
- 1/4 cup grated cheese (cheddar or feta)
- 1 tablespoon olive oil

- 2 tablespoons chopped fresh herbs (such as parsley or cilantro)
- Salt and pepper to taste

Instructions

1. Preheat your oven to 375°F (190°C).
2. In a skillet, sauté diced onions in olive oil until translucent.
3. Add bell peppers and callaloo, cooking until wilted.
4. In a bowl, whisk together eggs, salt, and pepper.
5. Pour the egg mixture into the skillet with the vegetables.
6. Sprinkle diced tomatoes, grated cheese, and chopped herbs evenly over the eggs.
7. Cook on the stovetop for a few minutes until the edges begin to set.
8. Transfer the skillet to the preheated oven and bake for about 15 minutes or until the frittata is cooked through and lightly browned on top.
9. Slice into wedges and serve.

Nutritional Values (per serving)

- Calories: 200 kcal
- Protein: 14g
- Carbohydrates: 5g
- Dietary Fiber: 2g
- Sugars: 2g
- Fat: 14g
- Saturated Fat: 4g
- Cholesterol: 330mg
- Sodium: 250mg

Cottage Cheese Toast

Prep Time: 5 minutes
Total Time: 5 minutes
Servings: 1

Ingredients

- 2 slices whole grain bread, toasted
- 1/2 cup low-fat cottage cheese
- 1/2 avocado, sliced
- 1 medium tomato, sliced
- Sprinkle of black pepper
- Optional: a drizzle of olive oil or balsamic glaze

Instructions

1. Toast the whole grain bread slices to your liking.
2. Spread an even layer of low-fat cottage cheese on each slice.
3. Top with avocado slices and tomato slices.

4. Sprinkle it with black pepper.
5. Optionally, drizzle with a bit of olive oil or balsamic glaze.

Nutritional Values (per serving)
- Calories: 350 kcal
- Protein: 20g
- Carbohydrates: 30g
- Dietary Fiber: 10g
- Sugars: 5g
- Fat: 18g
- Saturated Fat: 3g
- Cholesterol: 10mg
- Sodium: 450mg

Quinoa Breakfast Bowl with Scrambled Eggs & Veggies

Prep Time: 15 minutes
Cook Time: 20 minutes
Total Time: 35 minutes
Servings: 2

Ingredients
- 1/2 cup quinoa, rinsed
- 1 cup water or vegetable broth
- 4 large eggs, beaten
- 1 tablespoon olive oil
- 1/2 cup diced bell peppers (any color)
- 1/2 cup cherry tomatoes, halved
- 1/4 cup diced red onions
- 1/2 cup chopped spinach
- Salt and pepper to taste
- Optional toppings: avocado slices, hot sauce

Instructions
1. In a saucepan, combine quinoa and water or vegetable broth. Bring to a boil, then reduce heat, cover, and simmer for 15 minutes or until quinoa is cooked.
2. In a skillet over medium heat, heat the olive oil. Sauté the diced onions until they are transparent.
3. Add bell peppers, cherry tomatoes, and chopped spinach to the skillet. Cook until vegetables are tender.
4. Push the veggies to the side of the skillet, pour beaten eggs into the empty side, and scramble until cooked.
5. Mix the scrambled eggs with the vegetables. Season with salt and pepper.

6. Divide the cooked quinoa between two bowls and top with the egg and veggie mixture.
7. Add optional toppings such as avocado slices and hot sauce.

Nutritional Values (per serving
- Calories: 400 kcal
- Protein: 20g
- Carbohydrates: 40g
- Dietary Fiber: 7g
- Sugars: 4g
- Fat: 18g
- Saturated Fat: 4g
- Cholesterol: 370mg
- Sodium: 180mg

Frittata with Asparagus & Feta Cheese

Prep Time: 10 minutes
Cook Time: 20 minutes
Total Time: 30 minutes
Servings: 4

Ingredients
- 6 large eggs
- 1/2 bunch asparagus, trimmed and sliced into 1-inch segments
- 1/2 cup crumbled feta cheese
- 1/4 cup diced red onions
- 2 tablespoons olive oil
- 2 tablespoons chopped fresh dill
- Salt and pepper to taste

Instructions
1. Preheat your oven to 375°F (190°C).
2. In an oven-safe skillet, sauté diced red onions and asparagus in olive oil until asparagus is tender.
3. In a bowl, whisk together eggs, feta cheese, chopped dill, salt, and pepper.
4. Pour the egg mixture over the asparagus and onions in the skillet.
5. Cook on the stovetop for a few minutes until the edges begin to set.
6. Transfer the skillet to the preheated oven and bake for about 15 minutes or until the frittata is cooked through and lightly browned on top.
7. Slice into wedges and serve.

Nutritional Values (per serving)
- Calories: 220 kcal
- Protein: 14g
- Carbohydrates: 4g
- Dietary Fiber: 1g
- Sugars: 2g
- Fat: 16g
- Saturated Fat: 5g
- Cholesterol: 330mg
- Sodium: 340mg

Eggs, Toast & Strawberries

Prep Time: 10 minutes
Cook Time: 5 minutes
Total Time: 15 minutes
Servings: 2

Ingredients
- 4 large eggs
- 4 slices whole grain bread, toasted
- 1 cup fresh strawberries, sliced
- Butter or olive oil for cooking eggs
- Salt and pepper to taste

Instructions
1. In a skillet, heat butter or olive oil over medium heat.
2. Crack eggs into the skillet and cook to your liking (fried, scrambled, or poached).
3. Season eggs with salt and pepper.
4. Toast whole grain bread slices until golden brown.
5. Place the cooked eggs on the toast.
6. Serve with fresh strawberry slices on the side.

Nutritional Values (per serving)
- Calories: 350 kcal
- Protein: 18g
- Carbohydrates: 35g
- Dietary Fiber: 8g
- Sugars: 8g
- Fat: 16g
- Saturated Fat: 5g
- Cholesterol: 380mg
- Sodium: 450mg

Spinach & Feta Omelette

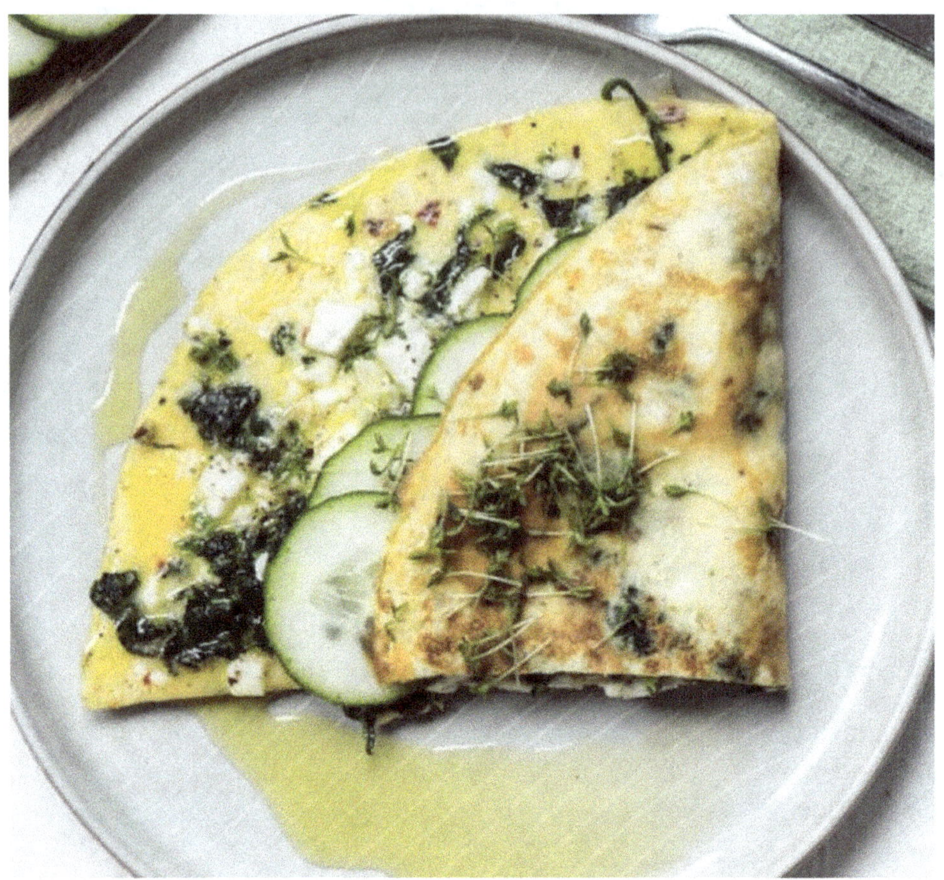

Prep Time: 10 minutes
Cook Time: 5 minutes
Total Time: 15 minutes
Servings: 1

Ingredients
- 2 large eggs
- 1 cup fresh spinach, chopped
- 2 tablespoons crumbled feta cheese
- 1/4 cup diced tomatoes
- 1/4 cup diced red onions
- 1 tablespoon olive oil
- Salt and pepper to taste
- Fresh herbs for garnish (optional)

Instructions
1. In a bowl, whisk together eggs until well combined.
2. In a non-stick skillet, heat the olive oil over medium heat
3. Add diced red onions and sauté until translucent.

4. Add chopped spinach to the skillet and cook until wilted.
5. Pour the whisked eggs over the spinach and onions.
6. Allow the eggs to set slightly at the edges, then gently lift the edges with a spatula to let the uncooked eggs flow underneath.
7. Sprinkle diced tomatoes and crumbled feta cheese evenly over one half of the omelette.
8. Fold the other half of the omelette over the filling.
9. Cook for an additional minute until the cheese is melted and the omelette is cooked through.
10. Season with salt and pepper, garnish with fresh herbs if desired, and serve.

Nutritional Values (per serving)
- Calories: 350 kcal
- Protein: 20g
- Carbohydrates: 8g
- Dietary Fiber: 2g
- Sugars: 3g
- Fat: 25g
- Saturated Fat: 7g
- Cholesterol: 385mg
- Sodium: 450mg

Cottage Cheese, Egg, Avocado Toast

Prep Time: 10 minutes
Cook Time: 5 minutes
Total Time: 15 minutes
Servings: 1

Ingredients
- 2 slices whole grain bread, toasted
- 1/2 cup low-fat cottage cheese
- 1 boiled egg, sliced
- 1/2 avocado, sliced
- Salt and pepper to taste
- A sprinkle of red pepper flakes or paprika (if preferred)

Instructions
1. Toast the whole grain bread slices to your liking.
2. Spread an even layer of low-fat cottage cheese on each slice.
3. Arrange sliced boiled egg and avocado on top of the cottage cheese.
4. Season with salt and pepper.
5. Optionally, sprinkle with red pepper flakes or paprika for extra flavor.

Nutritional Values (per serving)
- Calories: 400 kcal
- Protein: 25g
- Carbohydrates: 35g
- Dietary Fiber: 12g
- Sugars: 4g
- Fat: 20g
- Saturated Fat: 4g
- Cholesterol: 210mg
- Sodium: 400mg

Healthy Zucchini Bread

Prep Time: 15 minutes
Cook Time: 50 minutes
Total Time: 1 hour and 5 minutes
Servings: 12 slices

Ingredients
- 2 cups grated zucchini (about 2 medium-sized zucchinis)
- 2 cups whole wheat flour
- 1/2 cup coconut oil, melted
- 1/2 cup honey or maple syrup
- 2 large eggs
- 1 teaspoon vanilla extract
- 1 teaspoon cinnamon
- 1/2 teaspoon baking powder
- 1/2 teaspoon baking soda
- 1/4 teaspoon salt
- 1/2 cup chopped nuts (walnuts or almonds), optional

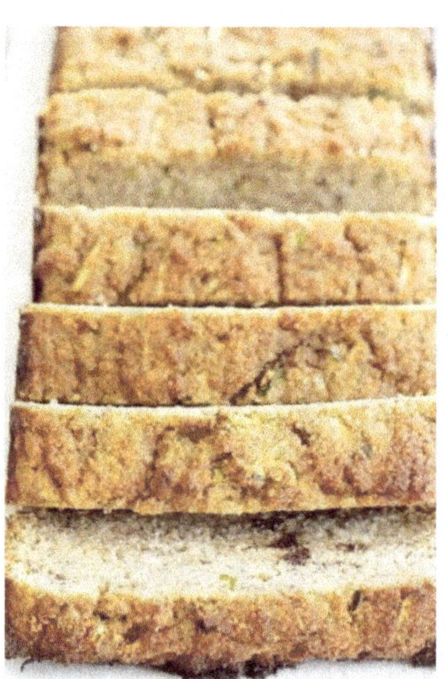

Instructions
1. Preheat the oven to 350°F (175°C) and grease a loaf pan with cooking spray
2. Grate the zucchinis and squeeze out excess moisture with a clean kitchen towel.
3. In a large bowl, whisk together melted coconut oil, honey or maple syrup, eggs, and vanilla extract.
4. Add grated zucchini to the wet ingredients and mix well.
5. In a separate bowl, combine whole wheat flour, cinnamon, baking powder, baking soda, and salt.
6. Add the dry ingredients to the wet ingredients while stirring until mixed.
7. If using, fold in chopped nuts.

8. After filling the loaf pan, level the top of the batter.
9. In order to ensure that a toothpick inserted into the centre comes out clean, bake for 50 to 60 minutes.
10. Allow the zucchini bread to cool in the pan for 10 minutes before transferring it to a wire rack to cool completely.

Nutritional Values (per slice)
- Calories: 200 kcal
- Protein: 4g
- Carbohydrates: 25g
- Dietary Fiber: 3g
- Sugars: 10g
- Fat: 11g
- Saturated Fat: 8g
- Cholesterol: 30mg
- Sodium: 120mg

Italian Eggs

Prep Time: 10 minutes
Cook Time: 10 minutes
Total Time: 20 minutes
Servings: 2

Ingredients
- 4 large eggs
- 1 cup cherry tomatoes, halved
- 1/4 cup diced red onions
- 2 cloves garlic, minced
- 1/4 cup fresh basil, chopped
- 2 tablespoons olive oil
- Salt and pepper to taste
- Grated Parmesan cheese for topping (optional)

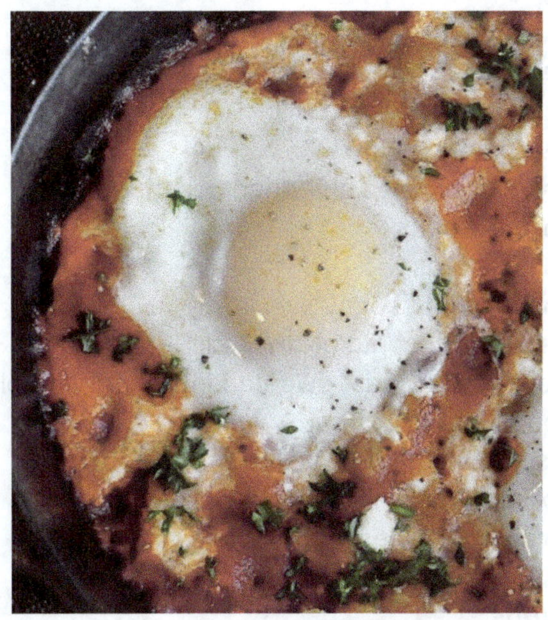

Instructions
1. In a skillet, heat olive oil over medium heat.
2. Add diced red onions and minced garlic, sauté until fragrant.
3. Cook the cherry tomatoes in the skillet until they begin to soften.
4. Create small wells in the tomato mixture and crack the eggs into each well.
5. Cover the skillet and cook until the egg whites are set but the yolks are still runny, or to your desired doneness.
6. Season with salt and pepper.

7. Sprinkle chopped fresh basil over the eggs.
8. Optionally, top with grated Parmesan cheese.

Nutritional Values (per serving)
- Calories: 250 kcal
- Protein: 12g
- Carbohydrates: 8g
- Dietary Fiber: 2g
- Sugars: 4g
- Fat: 18g
- Saturated Fat: 4g
- Cholesterol: 370mg
- Sodium: 160mg

Low-carb Granola with Greek Yogurt

Prep Time: 10 minutes
Cook Time: 20 minutes
Total Time: 30 minutes
Servings: 4

Ingredients
- 1 cup almonds, chopped
- 1 cup walnuts, chopped
- 1/2 cup unsweetened shredded coconut
- 1/4 cup chia seeds
- 1/4 cup flaxseeds
- 1/4 cup pumpkin seeds
- 2 tablespoons coconut oil, melted
- 2 tablespoons low-carb sweetener (e.g., erythritol or stevia)
- 1 teaspoon vanilla extract
- 1/2 teaspoon cinnamon
- Pinch of salt
- Greek yogurt for serving

Instructions
1. Preheat your oven to 300°F (150°C) and line a baking sheet with parchment paper.
2. In a large bowl, combine chopped almonds, chopped walnuts, shredded coconut, chia seeds, flaxseeds, and pumpkin seeds.
3. In a separate bowl, mix melted coconut oil, low-carb sweetener, vanilla extract, cinnamon, and a pinch of salt.
4. Pour the wet mixture over the dry ingredients and toss until well combined.
5. Spread the granola mixture evenly on the prepared baking sheet.

6. Bake for about 20 minutes or until golden brown, stirring halfway through to ensure even baking.
7. Allow the granola to cool completely before serving.
8. Serve with Greek yogurt.

Nutritional Values (per serving - granola only)
- Calories: 300 kcal
- Protein: 9g
- Carbohydrates: 10g
- Dietary Fiber: 6g
- Sugars: 2g
- Fat: 26g
- Saturated Fat: 8g
- Cholesterol: 0mg
- Sodium: 50mg

Broccoli & Cheese Crustless Quiche

Prep Time: 15 minutes
Cook Time: 40 minutes
Total Time: 55 minutes
Servings: 6

Ingredients
- 2 cups steamed and chopped broccoli florets
- 1 cup shredded cheddar cheese
- 1/2 cup diced onions
- 1/2 cup chopped (any colour) bell peppers
- 6 large eggs
- 1 cup milk (any type - almond, soy, or regular)
- 1 teaspoon Dijon mustard
- Salt and pepper to taste
- Greasing with olive oil or cooking spray

Instructions
1. Preheat your oven to 350°F (175°C) and grease a pie dish with olive oil or cooking spray.
2. Spread steamed and chopped broccoli evenly in the pie dish.
3. Sprinkle shredded cheddar cheese over the broccoli.
4. In a bowl, whisk together eggs, milk, Dijon mustard, salt, and pepper.
5. Add diced onions and bell peppers to the egg mixture and mix well.
6. Pour the egg mixture over the broccoli and cheese in the pie dish.
7. Bake for approximately 40 minutes or until the quiche is set and lightly browned on top.
8. Allow it to cool for a few minutes before slicing.

Nutritional Value
- Calories: 180 kcal
- Protein: 12g
- Carbohydrates: 6g
- Dietary Fiber: 2g
- Sugars: 3g
- Fat: 12g
- Saturated Fat: 5g
- Cholesterol: 210mg
- Sodium: 260mg

Avocado Egg Bacon Toast

Prep Time: 10 minutes
Cook Time: 10 minutes
Total Time: 20 minutes
Servings: 2
Ingredients
- 2 slices whole grain bread, toasted
- 1 ripe avocado, mashed
- 2 large eggs
- 2 slices cooked bacon
- Salt and pepper to taste
- Optional toppings: red pepper flakes, chopped chives

Instructions
1. Toast the whole grain bread slices to your liking.
2. Mash the ripe avocado and spread it evenly on the toasted bread.
3. Cook the eggs to your preference (poached, fried, or scrambled).
4. Place the cooked eggs on top of the mashed avocado.
5. Lay a slice of cooked bacon over each egg.
6. Season with salt and pepper.
7. Optionally, sprinkle with red pepper flakes or chopped chives for extra flavor.

Nutritional Values (per serving)
- Calories: 350 kcal
- Protein: 15g
- Carbohydrates: 25g
- Dietary Fiber: 8g
- Sugars: 2g
- Fat: 22g
- Saturated Fat: 5g
- Sodium: 450mg

Bacon & Brie Tortillas

Prep Time: 15 minutes
Cook Time: 10 minutes
Total Time: 25 minutes
Servings: 2

Ingredients
- 4 small whole wheat or corn tortillas
- 4 slices bacon, cooked and crumbled
- 4 oz Brie cheese, sliced
- 1 cup arugula or spinach
- 1 medium tomato, diced
- 1 tablespoon olive oil
- Salt and pepper to taste

Instructions
1. Heat the tortillas in a dry skillet or microwave until warmed.
2. In the same skillet, heat olive oil over medium heat.
3. Place Brie cheese slices on half of each tortilla.
4. Add crumbled bacon, diced tomatoes, and arugula or spinach on top of the Brie.
5. Fold the other half of the tortilla over the toppings, creating a semi-circle.
6. Cook each tortilla for about 2-3 minutes on each side or until the cheese is melted.
7. Season with salt and pepper to taste.

Nutritional Values (per serving - 2 tortillas)
- Calories: 500 kcal
- Protein: 20g
- Carbohydrates: 30g
- Dietary Fiber: 5g
- Sugars: 2g
- Fat: 35g
- Saturated Fat: 15g
- Cholesterol: 75mg
- Sodium: 500mg

Breakfast Pita Pocket

Prep Time: 10 minutes
Cook Time: 5 minutes
Total Time: 15 minutes
Servings: 2

Ingredients

- 2 whole wheat pita pockets
- 4 large eggs
- 1/2 cup chopped (any colour) bell peppers
- 1/4 cup diced onions
- 1/2 cup cherry tomatoes, halved
- 1/4 cup feta cheese, crumbled
- 1 tablespoon olive oil
- Salt and pepper to taste
- Fresh herbs for garnish (optional)

Instructions

1. Cut the whole wheat pita pockets in half to form pockets.
2. In a skillet, heat olive oil over medium heat.
3. Add diced onions and sauté until translucent.
4. Add diced bell peppers to the skillet and cook until slightly softened.
5. Crack eggs into the skillet and scramble until cooked.
6. Stir in halved cherry tomatoes and crumbled feta cheese.
7. Season with salt and pepper.
8. Spoon the egg mixture into the pita pockets.
9. Garnish with fresh herbs if desired.

Nutritional Values (per serving)

- Calories: 350 kcal
- Protein: 18g
- Carbohydrates: 30g
- Dietary Fiber: 6g
- Sugars: 4g
- Fat: 18g
- Saturated Fat: 5g
- Cholesterol: 370mg
- Sodium: 500mg

Coconut Flaxseed Porridge

Prep Time: 5 minutes
Cook Time: 10 minutes
Total Time: 15 minutes
Servings: 2

Ingredients

- 1/2 cup flax seeds
- 1 cup coconut milk

- 1 cup water
- 2 tablespoons unsweetened shredded coconut
- 1 tablespoon chia seeds
- 1 tablespoon honey or maple syrup (optional for sweetness)
- Toppings: fresh berries or sliced fruits

Instructions

1. In a saucepan, combine flaxseeds, coconut milk, and water.
2. Bring the mixture to a gentle simmer over medium heat, stirring continuously.
3. Add shredded coconut and chia seeds, continuing to stir.
4. Cook for about 5-7 minutes or until the porridge thickens to your desired consistency.
5. If desired, add honey or maple syrup for sweetness and mix well.
6. Remove from heat and let it cool slightly.
7. Serve the coconut flaxseed porridge in bowls, topped with fresh berries or sliced fruits.

Nutritional Values (per serving)

- Calories: 300 kcal
- Protein: 7g
- Carbohydrates: 20g
- Dietary Fiber: 12g
- Sugars: 5g
- Fat: 23g
- Saturated Fat: 13g
- Cholesterol: 0mg
- Sodium: 50mg

Apple Cinnamon Waffles

Prep Time: 15 minutes
Cook Time: 10 minutes
Total Time: 25 minutes
Servings: 4 (2 waffles each)

Ingredients

- 2 cups oat flour or almond flour
- 1 tablespoon baking powder
- 1 teaspoon ground cinnamon
- 1/2 teaspoon salt
- 1 3/4 cups unsweetened almond milk or any milk alternative
- 1/3 cup melted coconut oil or unsweetened applesauce
- 2 large eggs
- 1 teaspoon vanilla extract
- 1 peeled, cored, and coarsely chopped apple

1. Preheat your waffle maker per the manufacturer's directions.
2. In a large bowl, whisk together almond flour or oat flour, baking powder, ground cinnamon, and salt.
3. In another bowl, whisk together unsweetened almond milk or a milk alternative, melted coconut oil or unsweetened applesauce, eggs, and vanilla extract.
4. Stir the wet ingredients into the dry ingredients until they are solely mixed.
5. Gently fold in the finely chopped apple.
6. Lightly grease the waffle iron with non-stick cooking spray.
7. Pour the batter onto the preheated waffle iron and cook according to the manufacturer's instructions.
8. Repeat until all the batter is used.

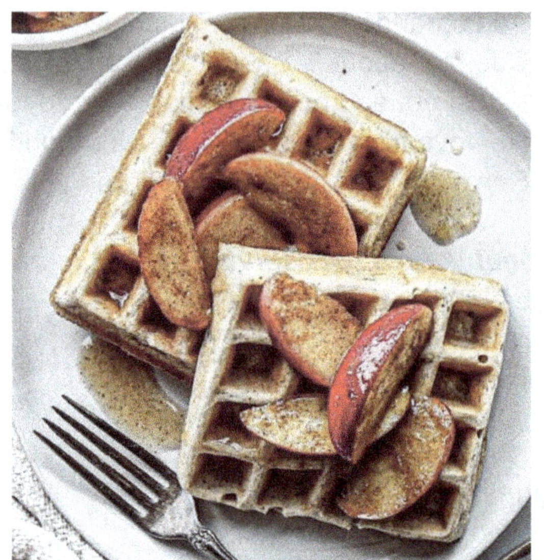

Nutritional Values (per serving - 2 waffles)

- Calories: 320 kcal
- Protein: 10g
- Carbohydrates: 15g
- Dietary Fiber: 5g
- Sugars: 2g
- Fat: 25g
- Saturated Fat: 10g
- Cholesterol: 60mg
- Sodium: 350mg

Bone Broth Poached Eggs

Prep Time: 5 minutes
Cook Time: 5 minutes
Total Time: 10 minutes
Servings: 2

Ingredients

- 4 large eggs
- 2 cups homemade or low-sodium store-bought bone broth
- 1 tablespoon white vinegar (optional)
- Salt and pepper to taste
- Chopped fresh herbs for garnish (optional)

Instructions

1. In a small saucepan, heat the bone broth over medium heat. If using, add white vinegar to the broth.
2. Bring the broth to a gentle simmer.

3. Crack each egg into a small bowl or ramekin.
4. Create a gentle whirlpool in the simmering broth using a spoon and carefully slide the eggs, one at a time, into the center of the whirlpool.
5. Poach the eggs for about 3-4 minutes for a soft yolk or longer if you prefer a firmer yolk.
6. Carefully remove the poached eggs with a slotted spoon and place them on a plate lined with paper towels to absorb excess broth.
7. Season with salt and pepper to taste.
8. Garnish with chopped fresh herbs if desired.

Nutritional Values (per serving)
- Calories: 150 kcal
- Protein: 15g
- Carbohydrates: 0g
- Dietary Fiber: 0g
- Sugars: 0g
- Fat: 10g
- Saturated Fat: 3g
- Cholesterol: 370mg
- Sodium: 200mg

Gestational Diabetes-Friendly Note: This recipe focuses on protein and is low in carbohydrates. Ensure the bone broth is low-sodium, and if you have concerns about vinegar, you can omit it without compromising the poaching process.

Grain Free Granolas

Prep Time: 10 minutes
Cook Time: 20 minutes
Total Time: 30 minutes
Servings: About 8 (1/2 cup each)

Ingredients
- 1 cup almonds, chopped
- 1 cup walnuts, chopped
- 1/2 cup unsweetened shredded coconut
- 1/4 cup sunflower seeds
- 1/4 cup pumpkin seeds
- 2 tablespoons chia seeds
- 2 tablespoons coconut oil, melted
- 2 tablespoons honey or maple syrup (optional for sweetness)
- 1 teaspoon vanilla extract
- 1/2 teaspoon ground cinnamon
- Pinch of salt
- 1/2 cup unsweetened dried fruits (e.g., cranberries, apricots, or raisins)

Instructions

1. Preheat your oven to 325°F (163°C) and line a baking sheet with parchment paper.
2. In a large bowl, combine chopped almonds, chopped walnuts, shredded coconut, sunflower seeds, pumpkin seeds, and chia seeds.
3. In a separate bowl, mix melted coconut oil, honey or maple syrup (if using), vanilla extract, ground cinnamon, and a pinch of salt.
4. Pour the wet mixture over the dry ingredients and toss until well combined.
5. Spread the granola mixture evenly on the prepared baking sheet.
6. Bake for about 20 minutes, stirring halfway through to ensure even baking.
7. Remove from the oven when golden brown and let it cool completely.
8. Once cooled, mix in unsweetened dried fruits of your choice.

Nutritional Values (per 1/2 cup serving)

- Calories: 250 kcal
- Protein: 7g
- Carbohydrates: 10g
- Dietary Fiber: 5g
- Sugars: 4g
- Fat: 20g
- Saturated Fat: 6g
- Cholesterol: 0mg
- Sodium: 50mg

Egg Tortilla Wrap

Prep Time: 10 minutes
Cook Time: 5 minutes
Total Time: 15 minutes
Servings: 2 wraps

Ingredients

- 4 large eggs
- 2 whole wheat or low-carb tortillas
- 1/2 cup baby spinach leaves
- 1/4 cup diced tomatoes
- 1/4 cup diced bell peppers (any color)
- 2 tablespoons feta cheese, crumbled
- 1 tablespoon olive oil
- Salt and pepper to taste
- Salsa or hot sauce for serving (optional)

Instructions

1. In a bowl, beat the eggs and season with salt and pepper.
2. In a skillet over medium heat, heat the olive oil.
3. Pour the beaten eggs into the skillet and scramble until cooked through.
4. Lay out the tortillas and divide the scrambled eggs evenly between them.
5. Add baby spinach leaves, diced tomatoes, diced bell peppers, and crumbled feta cheese on top of the eggs.
6. Fold the sides of the tortillas and roll them into wraps.
7. Optional: Warm the wraps in the skillet for a minute on each side.
8. Serve with salsa or hot sauce if desired.

Nutritional Values (per wrap)

- Calories: 300 kcal
- Protein: 15g
- Carbohydrates: 20g
- Dietary Fiber: 5g
- Sugars: 2g
- Fat: 18g
- Saturated Fat: 5g
- Cholesterol: 380mg
- Sodium: 400mg

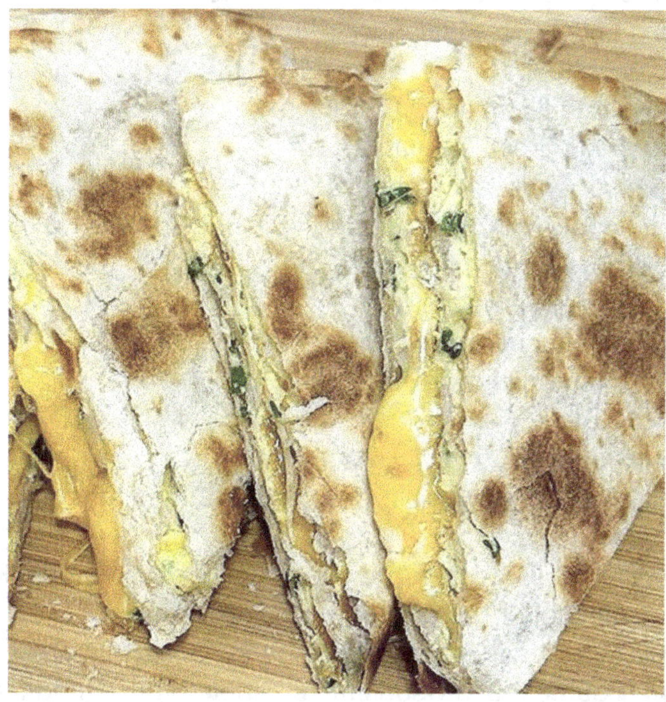

CHAPTER THREE: LUNCH AND DINNER RECIPES

Spicy Sweet Potato Soup

Prep Time: 15 minutes
Cook Time: 30 minutes
Total Time: 45 minutes
Servings: 4

Ingredients
- 2 large sweet potatoes, peeled and diced
- 1 tablespoon olive oil
- 1 onion, chopped
- 2 cloves garlic, minced
- 1 teaspoon ground cumin
- 1/2 teaspoon smoked paprika
- 1/4 teaspoon cayenne pepper (adjust to taste)
- 4 cups low-sodium vegetable broth
- Salt and pepper to taste
- 1/2 cup coconut milk (unsweetened)
- Fresh cilantro for garnish (optional)

Instruction
1. Heat the olive oil in a big pot over medium heat. Add chopped onions and cook until softened.
2. Add minced garlic, ground cumin, smoked paprika, and cayenne pepper. Stir for 1 minute, or until aromatic.
3. Add diced sweet potatoes to the pot and sauté for another 5 minutes.
4. Pour in the low-sodium vegetable broth. Bring the mixture to a boil, then lower to a low heat.
5. Cook until sweet potatoes are tender, about 20-25 minutes.
6. Puree the soup with an immersion blender until smooth. Alternatively, transfer the soup to a blender in batches.
7. Season with salt and pepper to taste.
8. Stir in coconut milk and heat through.
9. Garnish with fresh cilantro if desired.

Nutritional Values (per serving)
- Calories: 180 kcal
- Protein: 3g
- Carbohydrates: 30g

- Dietary Fiber: 4g
- Sugars: 8g
- Fat: 6g
- Saturated Fat: 3g
- Cholesterol: 0mg
- Sodium: 300mg

Salmon Miso Soup

Prep Time: 10 minutes
Cook Time: 15 minutes
Total Time: 25 minutes
Servings: 4

Ingredients
- 4 cups chicken or veggie broth (low sodium)
- 2 tablespoons miso paste (white or light)
- 1 cup shiitake mushrooms, sliced
- 1 cup baby spinach leaves
- 1 carrot, julienned
- 1 green onion, sliced
- 1/2 pound salmon fillet, skinless and boneless, cut into bite-sized pieces
- 1 tablespoon low-sodium soy sauce
- 1 teaspoon sesame oil
- 1 teaspoon grated ginger
- Optional: red pepper flakes for heat.

Instructions
1. In a pot, bring the low-sodium chicken or vegetable broth to a simmer.
2. In a small bowl, dissolve miso paste in a ladle of hot broth, then stir it back into the pot.
3. Add sliced shiitake mushrooms, julienned carrot, and salmon pieces to the pot.
4. Simmer for about 10 minutes until the salmon is cooked through.
5. Stir in baby spinach leaves until wilted.
6. Add low-sodium soy sauce, sesame oil, and grated ginger. You can adjust the flavour to your liking.
7. If desired, add red pepper flakes for some heat.
8. Garnish with sliced green onions.

Nutritional Values (per serving)
- Calories: 200 kcal
- Protein: 20g
- Carbohydrates: 10g
- Dietary Fiber: 2g

- Sugars: 3g
- Fat: 9g
- Saturated Fat: 1.5g
- Cholesterol: 40mg
- Sodium: 600mg

Cauliflower Leek Soup

Prep Time: 15 minutes
Cook Time: 25 minutes
Total Time: 40 minutes
Servings: 4

Ingredients
- 1 large cauliflower head, chopped into florets
- 2 sliced leeks, white and light green parts only
- 1 onion, chopped
- 2 cloves garlic, minced
- 4 cups low-sodium vegetable broth
- 1 tablespoon olive oil
- 1/2 teaspoon dried thyme
- Salt and pepper to taste
- 1 cup unsweetened almond milk or any milk alternative
- Chopped fresh chives for garnish (optional)

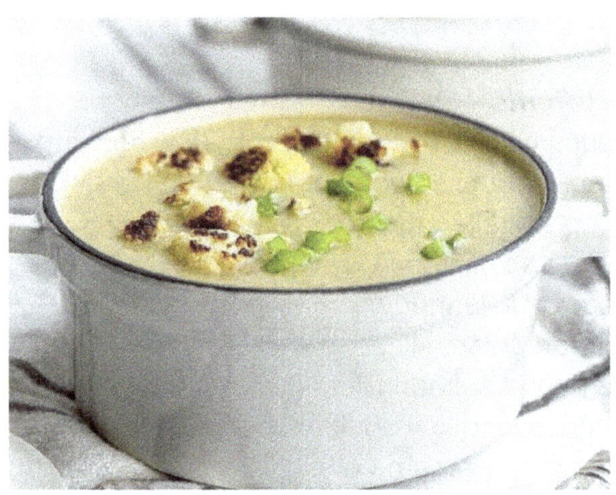

Instructions
1. Heat the olive oil in a big pot over medium heat. Add chopped onions, leeks, and garlic. Sauté until softened.
2. Add cauliflower florets to the pot and stir.
3. Pour in the low-sodium vegetable broth and add dried thyme.
4. Bring the mixture to a boil, then reduce to a simmer. Cook until the cauliflower is tender, about 20 minutes.
5. Puree the soup with an immersion blender until smooth. Alternatively, transfer the soup to a blender in batches.
6. Season to taste with salt and pepper.
7. Add unsweetened almond milk and heat through.
8. Garnish with chopped fresh chives if desired.

Nutritional Values (per serving)
- Calories: 120 kcal
- Protein: 4g
- Carbohydrates: 15g

- Dietary Fiber: 5g
- Sugars: 5g
- Fat: 6g
- Saturated Fat: 0.5g
- Cholesterol: 0mg
- Sodium: 400mg

Tuscan White Bean Soup

Prep Time: 15 minutes
Cook Time: 30 minutes
Total Time: 45 minutes
Servings: 4

Ingredients
- 2 cannellini beans (15 oz each), drained and washed
- 1 tablespoon olive oil
- 1 onion, finely chopped
- 2 carrots, diced
- 2 celery stalks, diced
- 3 cloves garlic, minced
- 1 teaspoon dried rosemary
- 1 teaspoon dried thyme
- 4 cups low-sodium vegetable broth
- 1 can (14 oz) undrained diced tomatoes
- 2 cups baby spinach leaves
- Salt and pepper to taste
- Grated Parmesan cheese for garnish (optional)

Instructions
1. Heat the olive oil in a big pot over medium heat. Add chopped onions, carrots, and celery. Sauté until softened.
2. Add minced garlic, dried rosemary, and dried thyme. Stir for about 1 minute until aromatic..
3. Pour in low-sodium vegetable broth, cannellini beans, and diced tomatoes (with their juices).
4. Bring the mixture to a boil, then reduce to a simmer. Cook for about 20 minutes.
5. Stir in baby spinach leaves until wilted.
6. To taste, season with salt and pepper.
7. Optional: Garnish with grated Parmesan cheese before serving.

Nutritional Values (per serving)
- Calories: 250 kcal
- Protein: 10g

- Carbohydrates: 40g
- Dietary Fiber: 10g
- Sugars: 4g
- Fat: 5g
- Saturated Fat: 0.5g
- Cholesterol: 0mg
- Sodium: 600mg

Lentil Soup

Prep Time: 15 minutes
Cook Time: 30 minutes
Total Time: 45 minutes
Servings: 4

Ingredients
- 1 cup dried green or brown lentils, rinsed
- 1 tablespoon olive oil
- 1 onion, finely chopped
- 2 carrots, diced
- 2 celery stalks, diced
- 3 cloves garlic, minced
- 1 teaspoon ground cumin
- 1 teaspoon ground coriander
- 6 cups low-sodium vegetable broth
- 1 can (14 oz) undrained diced tomatoes
- 2 cups chopped kale or spinach
- Salt and pepper to taste
- Lemon wedges for serving (optional)

Instructions
1. Heat the olive oil in a big pot over medium heat. Add chopped onions, carrots, and celery. Sauté until softened.
2. Add minced garlic, ground cumin, and ground coriander. Stir for 1 minute, or until aromatic.
3. Pour in low-sodium vegetable broth, lentils, and diced tomatoes (with their juices).
4. Bring the mixture to a boil, then reduce to a simmer. Cook for about 25 minutes or until lentils are tender.
5. Stir in chopped kale or spinach until wilted.
6. To taste, season with salt and pepper.
7. Optional: Serve with a squeeze of fresh lemon juice.

Nutritional Values (per serving)
- Calories: 300 kcal

- Protein: 18g
- Carbohydrates: 30g
- Dietary Fiber: 18g
- Sugars: 6g
- Fat: 3g
- Saturated Fat: 0.5g
- Cholesterol: 0mg
- Sodium: 600mg

Veggie Wrap

Prep Time: 15 minutes
Total Time: 15 minutes
Servings: 2 wraps

Ingredients
- 2 whole wheat or low-carb tortillas
- 1 cup baby spinach leaves
- 1/2 cup cucumber, thinly sliced
- 1/2 cup bell peppers (any color), thinly sliced
- 1/2 cup cherry tomatoes, halved
- 1/4 cup avocado, sliced
- 2 tablespoons hummus (low-carb or homemade)
- 1 tablespoon olive oil
- Salt and pepper to taste

Instructions
1. Lay out the tortillas on a flat surface.
2. Spread a tablespoon of hummus on each tortilla.
3. Layer baby spinach leaves, thinly sliced cucumber, bell peppers, cherry tomatoes, and avocado on each tortilla.
4. Drizzle olive oil over the veggies, and sprinkle with salt and pepper to taste.
5. Carefully fold the sides of the tortillas and roll them into wraps.
6. Optional: Secure with toothpicks if needed.

Nutritional Values (per wrap)
- Calories: 250 kcal
- Protein: 6g
- Carbohydrates: 25g
- Dietary Fiber: 8g
- Sugars: 3g
- Fat: 15g
- Saturated Fat: 2g
- Cholesterol: 0mg
- Sodium: 350mg

Lettuce Wrap

Prep Time: 15 minutes
Total Time: 15 minutes
Servings: 2 wraps

Ingredients
- 8 large lettuce leaves (e.g., iceberg or romaine)
- 1/2 pound ground turkey or chicken, lean
- 1 tablespoon olive oil
- 1/2 cup sliced bell peppers (any color)
- 1/2 cup cherry tomatoes, diced
- 1/4 cup red onion, finely chopped
- 1 clove garlic, minced
- 1 teaspoon ground cumin
- 1 teaspoon paprika
- Salt and pepper to taste
- 1/4 cup Greek yogurt or sour cream (optional for topping)

Instructions
1. In a skillet, heat olive oil over medium heat. Add lean ground turkey or chicken and cook until browned.
2. Add diced bell peppers, cherry tomatoes, red onion, minced garlic, ground cumin, paprika, salt, and pepper to the skillet. Cook until vegetables are tender.
3. Drain any excess liquid from the skillet if needed.
4. Lay out the large lettuce leaves on a flat surface.
5. Spoon the cooked ground meat and vegetable mixture onto each lettuce leaf.
6. Optional: Top with a dollop of Greek yogurt or sour cream.
7. Carefully fold the sides of the lettuce leaves and roll them into wraps.

Nutritional Values (per wrap)
- Calories: 200 kcal
- Protein: 20g
- Carbohydrates: 10g
- Dietary Fiber: 3g
- Sugars: 4g
- Fat: 8g
- Saturated Fat: 2g
- Cholesterol: 50mg
- Sodium: 200mg

Turkey Wrap

Prep Time: 15 minutes
Total Time: 15 minutes
Servings: 2 wraps

Ingredients
- 2 whole wheat or low-carb tortillas
- 1/2 pound lean ground turkey
- 1 tablespoon olive oil
- 1/2 cup cucumber, thinly sliced
- 1/2 cup cherry tomatoes, halved
- 1/4 cup red onion, finely chopped
- 1/4 cup feta cheese, crumbled (optional)
- 2 tbsp Greek yogurt (or sour cream)
- 1 tablespoon fresh dill, chopped
- Salt and pepper to taste

Instructions
1. In a skillet, heat olive oil over medium heat. Add lean ground turkey and cook until browned.
2. Add thinly sliced cucumber, cherry tomatoes, red onion, and crumbled feta cheese (if using) to the skillet. Cook, stirring occasionally, until the vegetables are soft.
3. In a small bowl, mix Greek yogurt or sour cream with fresh dill.
4. Lay out the tortillas on a flat surface.
5. Spoon the cooked turkey and vegetable mixture onto each tortilla.
6. Drizzle the Greek yogurt or sour cream mixture over the filling.
7. Season with salt and pepper to taste.
8. Carefully fold the sides of the tortillas and roll them into wraps.

Nutritional Values (per wrap)
- Calories: 300 kcal
- Protein: 20g
- Carbohydrates: 25g
- Dietary Fiber: 4g
- Sugars: 4g
- Fat: 14g
- Saturated Fat: 4g
- Cholesterol: 60mg
- Sodium: 400mg

Tuna or Salmon Sandwich

Prep Time: 10 minutes
Total Time: 10 minutes
Servings: 2 sandwiches

Ingredients
- 1 can (5 oz) tuna or salmon, drained
- 2 whole wheat bread slices or low-carb bread alternative
- 1/4 cup Greek yogurt or mayonnaise (sugar-free)
- 1 tablespoon Dijon mustard
- 1 celery stalk, finely chopped
- 1/4 cup cucumber, finely diced
- 1 tablespoon red onion, finely chopped
- Salt and pepper to taste
- Lettuce leaves for garnish
- Tomato slices for topping (optional)

Instructions
1. In a bowl, combine drained tuna or salmon, Greek yogurt or mayonnaise, Dijon mustard, chopped celery, diced cucumber, and chopped red onion.
2. Mix until all of the ingredients are equally combined.
3. Season with salt and pepper to taste.
4. Toast the whole wheat bread slices (if desired).
5. Spread the tuna or salmon mixture onto each bread slice.
6. Top with lettuce leaves and tomato slices (if using).
7. Optional: Add additional seasonings or herbs according to your preference.
8. Assemble the sandwiches and slice in half.

Nutritional Values (per sandwich)
- Calories: 250 kcal
- Protein: 20g
- Carbohydrates: 20g
- Dietary Fiber: 4g
- Sugars: 3g
- Fat: 10g
- Saturated Fat: 2g
- Cholesterol: 30mg
- Sodium: 400mg

Tuna or Salmon Salad

Prep Time: 15 minutes
Total Time: 15 minutes
Servings: 2 servings

Ingredients
- 1 can (5 oz) tuna or salmon, drained
- 2 cups mixed salad greens (e.g., spinach, arugula, or lettuce)
- 1/2 cucumber, sliced
- 1/2 cup cherry tomatoes, halved
- 1/4 cup red onion, thinly sliced
- 1/4 cup feta cheese, crumbled (optional)
- 2 tablespoons olive oil
- 1 tablespoon balsamic vinegar
- 1 teaspoon Dijon mustard
- Salt and pepper to taste
- Lemon wedges for serving (optional)

Instructions
1. In a bowl, combine drained tuna or salmon with mixed salad greens, sliced cucumber, cherry tomatoes, red onion, and crumbled feta cheese (if using).
2. In a small jar, whisk together olive oil, balsamic vinegar, Dijon mustard, salt, and pepper to create the dressing.
3. Pour the dressing over the salad and gently toss to coat.
4. Divide the salad into two servings.
5. Optional: Squeeze lemon wedges over the salad before serving.

Nutritional Values (per serving)
- Calories: 300 kcal
- Protein: 20g
- Carbohydrates: 15g
- Dietary Fiber: 4g
- Sugars: 6g
- Fat: 20g
- Saturated Fat: 4g
- Cholesterol: 30mg
- Sodium: 500mg

Easy Taco Salad

Prep Time: 15 minutes
Cook Time: 10 minutes
Total Time: 25 minutes
Servings: 2 servings

Ingredients

- 1/2 pound ground turkey or chicken, lean
- 1 tablespoon olive oil
- 1 teaspoon ground cumin
- 1 teaspoon chili powder
- 1/2 teaspoon paprika
- Salt and pepper to taste
- 2 cups mixed salad greens (lettuce, spinach, etc.)
- 1/2 cup cherry tomatoes, halved
- 1/4 cup black beans, drained and rinsed
- 1/4 cup corn kernels (fresh or frozen, thawed)
- 1/4 cup red onion, finely chopped
- 1/4 cup shredded cheddar cheese
- 1/4 cup salsa (sugar-free)
- 2 tbsp. Greek yogurt or sour cream
- Fresh cilantro for garnish (optional)
- Lime wedges for serving (optional)

Instructions

1. In a skillet, heat olive oil over medium heat. Add lean ground turkey or chicken and cook until browned.
2. Add ground cumin, chili powder, paprika, salt, and pepper to the skillet. Stir until well combined.
3. In a large bowl, combine mixed salad greens, cherry tomatoes, black beans, corn, red onion, and shredded cheddar cheese.
4. Add the cooked ground meat mixture to the salad bowl.
5. Drizzle salsa over the salad and toss gently to combine.
6. Divide the salad into two servings.
7. Top each serving with a dollop of Greek yogurt or sour cream.
8. Optional: Garnish with fresh cilantro and serve with lime wedges.

Nutritional Values (per serving)

- Calories: 350 kcal
- Protein: 25g
- Carbohydrates: 25g
- Dietary Fiber: 6g
- Sugars: 5g
- Fat: 18g
- Saturated Fat: 6g
- Sodium: 450mg

Crispy Buffalo Chicken Salad

Prep Time: 15 minutes
Cook Time: 15 minutes
Total Time: 30 minutes
Servings: 2 servings

Ingredients
For Crispy Chicken:
- 1/2 pound boneless, skinless chicken breasts
- 1/2 cup almond flour
- 1 teaspoon garlic powder
- 1 teaspoon paprika
- Salt and pepper to taste
- 1 large egg, beaten
- Cooking spray

For Salad:
- 4 cups mixed salad greens (lettuce, spinach, etc.)
- 1/2 cup cherry tomatoes, halved
- 1/4 cup cucumber, sliced
- 1/4 cup celery, sliced
- 1/4 cup blue cheese crumbles (optional)
- 2 tablespoons olive oil
- 2 tablespoons buffalo sauce (sugar-free)
- Greek yogurt or sour cream for dressing (optional)

Instructions
1. Preheat the oven to 400°F (200°C).
2. In a bowl, mix almond flour, garlic powder, paprika, salt, and pepper.
3. Dip each chicken breast into the beaten egg, then coat with the almond flour mixture.
4. Place the coated chicken breasts on a baking sheet sprayed with cooking spray.
5. Bake for 15-20 minutes or until the chicken is cooked through and crispy.
6. In a large bowl, combine mixed salad greens, cherry tomatoes, cucumber, celery, and blue cheese crumbles (if using).
7. Slice the crispy chicken and place it on top of the salad.
8. In a small bowl, whisk together olive oil and buffalo sauce. Drizzle over the salad.
9. Toss the salad gently to coat evenly.
10. Serve with a dollop of Greek yogurt or sour cream if desired.

Nutritional Values (per serving)
- Calories: 400 kcal
- Protein: 30g

- Carbohydrates: 15g
- Dietary Fiber: 6g
- Sugars: 3g
- Fat: 25g
- Saturated Fat: 5g
- Cholesterol: 120mg
- Sodium: 600mg

Panzanella Chicken Caesar Salad

Prep Time: 20 minutes
Cook Time: 15 minutes
Total Time: 35 minutes
Servings: 2 servings

Ingredients
For Grilled Chicken:
- 1/2 pound boneless, skinless chicken breasts
- 1 tablespoon olive oil
- 1 teaspoon Italian seasoning
- Salt and pepper to taste

For Panzanella Salad:
- 4 cups mixed salad greens (e.g., romaine lettuce, arugula)
- 1 cup cherry tomatoes, halved
- 1/2 cucumber, sliced
- 1/4 cup red onion, thinly sliced
- 1 cup whole grain or low-carb bread, cubed
- 1 tablespoon olive oil
- 1 teaspoon garlic powder
- Salt and pepper to taste

For Caesar Dressing:
- 2 tablespoons Greek yogurt or mayonnaise (sugar-free)
- 1 tablespoon Dijon mustard
- 1 tablespoon lemon juice
- 1 clove garlic, minced
- 1/4 cup grated Parmesan cheese
- Salt and pepper to taste

Instructions

1. Preheat the grill or grill pan.
2. In a bowl, mix olive oil, Italian seasoning, salt, and pepper. Coat the chicken breasts with this mixture.
3. Grill the chicken for about 6-8 minutes per side or until cooked through.
4. In a large bowl, combine mixed salad greens, cherry tomatoes, cucumber, and red onion.
5. Toss the bread cubes with olive oil, garlic powder, salt, and pepper. Toast them in a skillet until golden brown.
6. Slice the grilled chicken and add it to the salad.
7. In a small bowl, whisk together Greek yogurt or mayonnaise, Dijon mustard, lemon juice, minced garlic, Parmesan cheese, salt, and pepper to make the Caesar dressing.
8. Pour the Caesar dressing over the salad and toss gently.
9. Add the toasted bread cubes to the salad for a Panzanella touch.
10. Serve immediately.

Nutritional Values (per serving)
- Calories: 450 kcal
- Protein: 30g
- Carbohydrates: 25g
- Dietary Fiber: 6g
- Sugars: 5g
- Fat: 25g
- Saturated Fat: 5g
- Cholesterol: 80mg
- Sodium: 600mg

Fruit Chicken & Walnut Salad

Prep Time: 15 minutes
Cook Time: 15 minutes (if grilling chicken)
Total Time: 30 minutes
Servings: 2 servings

Ingredients
For Grilled Chicken:
- 1/2 pound boneless, skinless chicken breasts
- 1 tablespoon olive oil
- 1 teaspoon lemon zest
- 1 teaspoon dried oregano
- Salt and pepper to taste

For Salad:
- 4 cups mixed salad greens (e.g., spinach, arugula)

- 1 cup strawberries, sliced
- 1/2 cup blueberries
- 1/4 cup red onion, thinly sliced
- 1/4 cup walnuts, chopped and toasted

For Dressing:
- 2 tablespoons olive oil
- 1 tablespoon balsamic vinegar
- 1 teaspoon Dijon mustard
- 1 teaspoon honey or a sugar-free alternative
- Salt and pepper to taste

Instructions

1. Preheat the grill or grill pan.
2. In a bowl, mix olive oil, lemon zest, dried oregano, salt, and pepper. Coat the chicken breasts with this mixture.
3. Grill the chicken for about 6-8 minutes per side or until cooked through.
4. In a large bowl, combine mixed salad greens, sliced strawberries, blueberries, red onion, and toasted walnuts.
5. Slice the grilled chicken and add it to the salad.
6. In a small bowl, whisk together olive oil, balsamic vinegar, Dijon mustard, honey, salt, and pepper to make the dressing.
7. Drizzle the dressing over the salad and toss gently.
8. Serve immediately.

Nutritional Values (per serving)

- Calories: 400 kcal
- Protein: 25g
- Carbohydrates: 20g
- Dietary Fiber: 6g
- Sugars: 10g
- Fat: 25g
- Saturated Fat: 3g
- Cholesterol: 70mg
- Sodium: 200mg

Rotisserie Chicken Salad

Prep Time: 15 minutes
Total Time: 15 minutes
Servings: 2 servings

Ingredients
- 2 cups rotisserie chicken, shredded (skinless and boneless)
- 4 cups mixed salad greens (e.g., romaine lettuce, arugula)
- 1 cup cherry tomatoes, halved
- 1/2 cucumber, sliced
- 1/4 cup red onion, thinly sliced
- 1/4 cup feta cheese, crumbled (optional)
- 1/4 cup pitted and sliced Kalamata olives
- 2 tablespoons olive oil
- 1 tablespoon red wine vinegar
- 1 teaspoon Dijon mustard
- 1 teaspoon dried oregano
- Salt and pepper to taste
- Lemon wedges for serving (optional)

Instructions
1. In a large bowl, combine shredded rotisserie chicken, mixed salad greens, cherry tomatoes, sliced cucumber, red onion, feta cheese (if using), and sliced Kalamata olives.
2. In a small bowl, whisk together olive oil, red wine vinegar, Dijon mustard, dried oregano, salt, and pepper to create the dressing.
3. Pour the dressing over the salad and gently toss to coat.
4. Divide the salad into two servings.
5. Optional: Serve with lemon wedges for an extra burst of flavor.

Nutritional Values (per serving)
- Calories: 350 kcal
- Protein: 25g
- Carbohydrates: 10g
- Dietary Fiber: 4g
- Sugars: 4g
- Fat: 25g
- Saturated Fat: 5g
- Cholesterol: 80mg
- Sodium: 600mg

Grilled Blue Cheese Steak Salad

Prep Time: 15 minutes
Cook Time: 15 minutes
Total Time: 30 minutes
Servings: 2 servings

Ingredients

For Grilled Steak:
- 1/2 pound sirloin or flank steak
- 1 tablespoon olive oil
- 1 teaspoon garlic powder
- 1 teaspoon dried thyme
- Salt and pepper to taste

For Salad:
- 4 cups mixed salad greens (e.g., spinach, arugula)
- 1/2 cup cherry tomatoes, halved
- 1/4 cup red onion, thinly sliced
- 1/4 cup cucumber, sliced
- 1/4 cup blue cheese, crumbled
- 1/4 cup walnuts, chopped and toasted

For Dressing:
- 2 tablespoons olive oil
- 1 tablespoon balsamic vinegar
- 1 teaspoon Dijon mustard
- Salt and pepper to taste

Instructions

1. Preheat the grill or grill pan.
2. In a bowl, mix olive oil, garlic powder, dried thyme, salt, and pepper. Coat the steak with this mixture.
3. Grill the steak for about 5-7 minutes per side or until desired doneness.
4. In a large bowl, combine mixed salad greens, cherry tomatoes, red onion, sliced cucumber, blue cheese, and toasted walnuts.
5. Slice the grilled steak and place it on top of the salad.
6. In a small bowl, whisk together olive oil, balsamic vinegar, Dijon mustard, salt, and pepper to make the dressing.
7. Drizzle the dressing over the salad and toss gently.
8. Serve immediately.

Nutritional Values (per serving)

- Calories: 400 kcal
- Protein: 30g
- Carbohydrates: 10g
- Dietary Fiber: 4g
- Sugars: 3g
- Fat: 28g
- Saturated Fat: 7g
- Sodium: 400mg

Greek Potato Salad Recipe with Green Beans

Prep Time: 15 minutes
Cook Time: 15 minutes
Total Time: 30 minutes
Servings: 4 servings

Ingredients
- 4 medium-sized potatoes, cubed (preferably low glycemic index potatoes)
- 1 cup trimmed and sliced green beans into bite-sized pieces
- 1/4 cup red onion, finely chopped
- 1/4 cup pitted and sliced Kalamata olives
- 1/4 cup feta cheese, crumbled (optional)
- 2 tablespoons olive oil
- 1 tablespoon red wine vinegar
- 1 teaspoon Dijon mustard
- 1 teaspoon dried oregano
- Salt and pepper to taste
- Fresh parsley for garnish (optional)

Instructions
1. Boil the cubed potatoes in salted water until tender, about 10-12 minutes. In the last 3 minutes of cooking, add the green beans to the boiling water. Drain and let them cool.
2. In a large bowl, combine the cooked potatoes, green beans, red onion, Kalamata olives, and feta cheese (if using).
3. In a small bowl, whisk together olive oil, red wine vinegar, Dijon mustard, dried oregano, salt, and pepper to create the dressing.
4. Toss the salad lightly with the dressing to coat.
5. Garnish with fresh parsley if desired.
6. Serve at room temperature or chilled.

Nutritional Values (per serving)
- Calories: 250 kcal
- Protein: 5g
- Carbohydrates: 35g
- Dietary Fiber: 5g
- Sugars: 3g
- Fat: 10g
- Saturated Fat: 2g
- Cholesterol: 5mg
- Sodium: 300mg

Quinoa Arugula Salad with Lemon Vinaigrette

Prep Time: 15 minutes
Cook Time: 15 minutes
Total Time: 30 minutes
Servings: 4 servings

Ingredients

For Quinoa:
- 1 cup quinoa, rinsed
- 2 cups water
- 1/4 teaspoon salt

For Salad:
- 4 cups arugula, washed and dried
- 1/2 cup cherry tomatoes, halved
- 1/4 cup red onion, thinly sliced
- 1/4 cup feta cheese, crumbled (optional)
- 1/4 cup walnuts, chopped and toasted

For Lemon Vinaigrette:
- 3 tablespoons olive oil
- 2 tablespoons lemon juice
- 1 teaspoon Dijon mustard
- 1 teaspoon honey or a sugar-free alternative
- Salt and pepper to taste

Instructions
1. Combine the quinoa, water, and salt in a medium saucepan. Bring to a boil, then reduce to a low heat, cover, and cook for 15 minutes, or until the quinoa is tender and the water has been absorbed. Allow to cool after fluffing with a fork.
2. In a large bowl, combine cooked quinoa, arugula, cherry tomatoes, red onion, feta cheese (if using), and toasted walnuts.
3. In a small bowl, whisk together olive oil, lemon juice, Dijon mustard, honey, salt, and pepper to create the vinaigrette.
4. Pour the lemon vinaigrette over the salad and toss gently to coat.
5. Serve at room temperature or chilled.

Nutritional Values (per serving)
- Calories: 300 kcal
- Protein: 8g
- Carbohydrates: 30g

- Dietary Fiber: 5g
- Sugars: 3g
- Fat: 18g
- Saturated Fat: 2g
- Cholesterol: 5mg
- Sodium: 200mg

Chicken Stir fry

Prep Time: 15 minutes
Cook Time: 15 minutes
Total Time: 30 minutes
Servings: 4 servings

Ingredients
- 1 pound boneless, skinless chicken breasts, thinly sliced
- 2 tablespoons low-sodium soy sauce
- 1 tablespoon olive oil
- 1 tablespoon sesame oil
- 2 cloves garlic, minced
- 1 teaspoon ginger, grated
- 1 cup broccoli florets
- 1 cup bell peppers, thinly sliced
- 1 cup snap peas, trimmed
- 1 medium carrot, julienned
- 1 tablespoon cornstarch
- 1/4 cup water
- Sesame seeds for garnish (optional)
- Green onions, sliced for garnish (optional)

Instructions:
1. In a bowl, marinate the sliced chicken in low-sodium soy sauce for 10 minutes.
2. In a large wok or skillet, heat olive oil and sesame oil over medium-high heat.
3. Add minced garlic and grated ginger, sautéing for 30 seconds until fragrant.
4. Add the marinated chicken to the wok and stir-fry until browned and cooked through.
5. Push the cooked chicken to the side of the wok. Add broccoli, bell peppers, snap peas, and julienned carrot. Stir-fry the vegetables until they are crisp-tender.
6. In a small bowl, mix cornstarch with water to create a slurry. Pour the slurry over the stir fry and toss to coat, allowing the sauce to thicken.
7. Garnish with sesame seeds and sliced green onions if desired.
8. Serve over cauliflower rice or a small portion of brown rice.

Nutritional Values (per serving)
- Calories: 250 kcal

- Protein: 25g
- Carbohydrates: 15g
- Dietary Fiber: 4g
- Sugars: 5g
- Fat: 10g
- Saturated Fat: 2g
- Cholesterol: 60mg
- Sodium: 500mg

Chicken & Vegetable Kebab

Prep Time: 20 minutes
Marinating Time: 30 minutes
Cook Time: 15 minutes
Total Time: 1 hour 5 minutes
Servings: 4 servings

Ingredients
For Marinade:
- 1 pound boneless, skinless chicken breasts, cut into cubes
- 2 tablespoons olive oil
- 1 tablespoon lemon juice
- 2 cloves garlic, minced
- 1 teaspoon dried oregano
- Salt and pepper to taste

For Kebabs:
- 1 bell pepper, cut into chunks
- 1 zucchini, sliced
- 1 red onion, cut into wedges
- Cherry tomatoes
- Wooden or metal skewers

Instructions
1. In a bowl, combine olive oil, lemon juice, minced garlic, dried oregano, salt, and pepper for the marinade.
2. Add chicken cubes to the marinade, ensuring they are well-coated. Marinate in the refrigerator for at least 30 minutes.
3. Preheat the grill or grill pan.
4. Thread marinated chicken, bell pepper chunks, zucchini slices, red onion wedges, and cherry tomatoes onto skewers, alternating between ingredients.
5. Grill the kebabs for about 12-15 minutes, turning occasionally, until the chicken is cooked through and vegetables are tender.
6. Serve the kebabs with a side of Greek yogurt or a yogurt-based sauce.

Nutritional Values (per serving)
- Calories: 250 kcal
- Protein: 25g
- Carbohydrates: 10g
- Dietary Fiber: 3g
- Sugars: 5g
- Fat: 12g
- Saturated Fat: 2g
- Cholesterol: 65mg
- Sodium: 300mg

Pepperoni Cauliflower Pizza

Prep Time: 15 minutes
Cook Time: 30 minutes
Total Time: 45 minutes
Servings: 4 servings

Ingredients
For Cauliflower Crust:
- 1 medium-sized cauliflower head, grated or processed into rice
- 1 egg
- 1/2 cup mozzarella cheese, shredded
- 1 teaspoon dried oregano
- 1/2 teaspoon garlic powder
- Salt and pepper to taste

For Toppings:
- 1/2 cup sugar-free pizza sauce
- 1 cup mozzarella cheese, shredded
- 1/2 cup sliced pepperoni (choose a low-carb and nitrate-free option)
- Fresh basil leaves for garnish (optional)

Instructions:
1. Preheat the oven to 425°F (220°C).
2. Microwave the grated cauliflower in a microwave-safe bowl for 5-6 minutes, or until soft. Let it cool.
3. Wrap the cooled cauliflower rice in a clean kitchen towel and squeeze out excess moisture.
4. In a bowl, combine cauliflower rice, egg, mozzarella cheese, dried oregano, garlic powder, salt, and pepper to create the crust mixture.
5. Line a baking sheet with parchment paper and spread the cauliflower mixture into a thin, round crust.
6. Bake the crust for 20-25 minutes or until golden brown and firm.

7. Remove the crust from the oven and spread sugar-free pizza sauce evenly.
8. Sprinkle shredded mozzarella cheese and top with sliced pepperoni.
9. Return the pizza to the oven for 10 minutes more, or until the cheese is melted and bubbling.
10. Garnish with fresh basil leaves if desired.

Nutritional Values (per serving)
- Calories: 200 kcal
- Protein: 15g
- Carbohydrates: 10g
- Dietary Fiber: 3g
- Sugars: 2g
- Fat: 12g
- Saturated Fat: 6g
- Cholesterol: 65mg
- Sodium: 500mg

Onion Mushroom Potato Pepper Steak Kabobs

Prep Time: 30 minutes
Marinating Time: 1 hour
Cook Time: 20 minutes
Total Time: 1 hour 50 minutes (including marinating)
Servings: 4 servings

Ingredients
For Marinade:
- 1 pound sirloin or flank steak, cut into cubes
- 2 tablespoons olive oil
- 2 tablespoons balsamic vinegar
- 2 cloves garlic, minced
- 1 teaspoon dried thyme
- Salt and pepper to taste

For Kabobs:
- 1 red onion, cut into wedges
- 1 cup mushrooms, cleaned and halved
- 1 cup baby potatoes, parboiled and halved
- 1 bell pepper, cut into chunks
- Wooden or metal skewers

Instructions
1. In a bowl, mix olive oil, balsamic vinegar, minced garlic, dried thyme, salt, and pepper for the marinade.

2. Add steak cubes to the marinade, ensuring they are well-coated. Marinate for at least 1 hour in the refrigerator.
3. Preheat the grill or grill pan.
4. Thread marinated steak, red onion wedges, mushrooms, baby potatoes, and bell pepper chunks onto skewers, alternating between ingredients.
5. Grill the kabobs for about 15-20 minutes, turning occasionally, until the steak reaches your desired doneness and vegetables are tender.
6. Serve the kabobs with a side of mixed greens or a low-carb dip.

Nutritional Values (per serving)
- Calories: 300 kcal
- Protein: 25g
- Carbohydrates: 15g
- Dietary Fiber: 3g
- Sugars: 3g
- Fat: 15g
- Saturated Fat: 4g
- Cholesterol: 60mg
- Sodium: 300mg

Chicken Drumsticks, Zucchini Fries, & Brown Rice

Prep Time: 20 minutes
Cook Time: 40 minutes
Total Time: 1 hour
Servings: 4 servings

Ingredients
For Chicken Drumsticks:
- 8 chicken drumsticks, skinless
- 2 tablespoons olive oil
- 1 teaspoon smoked paprika
- 1 teaspoon garlic powder
- 1 teaspoon onion powder
- Salt and pepper to taste

For Zucchini Fries:
- 2 medium-sized zucchini, cut into fries
- 2 tablespoons almond flour
- 1 teaspoon dried Italian herbs
- Salt and pepper to taste
- Cooking spray

For Brown Rice:
- 1 cup brown rice, uncooked
- 2 cups water
- Salt to taste

Instructions

1. Preheat the oven to 400°F (200°C).
2. In a bowl, mix olive oil, smoked paprika, garlic powder, onion powder, salt, and pepper. Coat the chicken drumsticks with this mixture.
3. Place the chicken drumsticks on a baking sheet lined with parchment paper and bake for 35-40 minutes or until golden brown and cooked through.
4. In a separate bowl, toss zucchini fries with almond flour, dried Italian herbs, salt, and pepper.
5. Arrange the coated zucchini fries on another baking sheet and spray them lightly with cooking spray.
6. Bake the zucchini fries for 20-25 minutes or until crispy and golden brown.
7. Meanwhile, cook brown rice in water with a pinch of salt according to package instructions.
8. Serve the chicken drumsticks, zucchini fries, and brown rice together.

Nutritional Values (per serving)
- Calories: 450 kcal
- Protein: 30g
- Carbohydrates: 40g
- Dietary Fiber: 5g
- Sugars: 2g
- Fat: 18g
- Saturated Fat: 4g
- Cholesterol: 90mg
- Sodium: 400mg

Turkey Burger & Sweet Potato Fries

Prep Time: 20 minutes
Cook Time: 30 minutes
Total Time: 50 minutes
Servings: 4 servings

Ingredients
For Turkey Burgers:
- 1 pound ground turkey, lean
- 1/4 cup almond flour
- 1 egg
- 1 teaspoon garlic powder

- 1 teaspoon onion powder
- 1 teaspoon dried oregano
- Salt and pepper to taste
- Lettuce leaves for wrapping

For Sweet Potato Fries:
- 2 large sweet potatoes, cut into fries
- 2 tablespoons olive oil
- 1 teaspoon smoked paprika
- 1/2 teaspoon garlic powder
- Salt and pepper to taste

Instructions

1. Preheat the oven to 425°F (220°C).
2. In a bowl, combine ground turkey, almond flour, egg, garlic powder, onion powder, dried oregano, salt, and pepper. Form into four burger patties.
3. Heat a grill pan or skillet over medium-high heat. Cook the turkey burgers for 5-6 minutes per side, or until done.
4. While burgers are cooking, toss sweet potato fries with olive oil, smoked paprika, garlic powder, salt, and pepper.
5. Spread sweet potato fries on a baking sheet lined with parchment paper and bake for 20-25 minutes or until golden and crispy.
6. Serve the turkey burgers wrapped in lettuce leaves and accompanied by sweet potato fries.

Nutritional Values (per serving)
- Calories: 350 kcal
- Protein: 25g
- Carbohydrates: 30g
- Dietary Fiber: 5g
- Sugars: 6g
- Fat: 15g
- Saturated Fat: 3g
- Cholesterol: 100mg
- Sodium: 400mg

Chicken Cheese Quesadilla

Prep Time: 15 minutes
Cook Time: 10 minutes
Total Time: 25 minutes
Servings: 2 servings

Ingredients
- 2 whole wheat or low-carb tortillas
- 1 cup cooked chicken breast, shredded
- 1/2 cup shredded low-fat cheddar or Monterey Jack cheese
- 1/4 cup diced tomatoes
- 1/4 cup diced bell peppers (use a variety of colors)
- 2 tablespoons diced red onion
- 1 tablespoon chopped fresh cilantro
- 1 teaspoon olive oil
- Guacamole and salsa for serving (optional)

Instructions
1. In a bowl, mix shredded chicken, cheese, diced tomatoes, diced bell peppers, red onion, and chopped cilantro.
2. In a skillet over medium heat, heat the olive oil.
3. Place one tortilla in the skillet and spread half of the chicken and vegetable mixture evenly over it.
4. Top with the second tortilla.
5. Cook for 3-4 minutes on each side or until the tortillas are golden brown, and the cheese is melted.
6. Remove from the skillet, let it cool for a minute, then cut into wedges.
7. Repeat the process for the second quesadilla.
8. If desired, top with guacamole and salsa.

Nutritional Values (per serving)
- Calories: 350 kcal
- Protein: 25g
- Carbohydrates: 25g
- Dietary Fiber: 5g
- Sugars: 2g
- Fat: 15g
- Saturated Fat: 5g
- Cholesterol: 60mg
- Sodium: 400mg

Peanut Zoodle

Prep Time: 15 minutes
Cook Time: 5 minutes
Total Time: 20 minutes
Servings: 2 servings

Ingredients

- 2 medium zucchinis, spiralized into zoodles
- 1/4 cup natural peanut butter (unsweetened)
- 2 tablespoons low-sodium soy sauce
- 1 tablespoon rice vinegar
- 1 tablespoon sesame oil
- 1 tablespoon grated ginger
- 1 clove garlic, minced
- 1 teaspoon chili flakes (optional)
- 1/4 cup chopped green onions
- 1/4 cup chopped peanuts for garnish

Instructions

1. Spiralize the zucchinis into zoodles using a spiralizer.
2. In a small bowl, whisk together peanut butter, soy sauce, rice vinegar, sesame oil, grated ginger, minced garlic, and chili flakes if desired.
3. Over medium heat, preheat a large skillet.
4. Add the zoodles to the skillet and toss for about 2-3 minutes until they are just tender.
5. Pour the peanut sauce over the zoodles and toss to coat evenly. Cook for an additional 2 minutes.
6. Remove from heat and garnish with chopped green onions and peanuts.
7. Serve immediately.

Nutritional Values (per serving)

- Calories: 300 kcal
- Protein: 10g
- Carbohydrates: 15g
- Dietary Fiber: 4g
- Sugars: 5g
- Fat: 25g
- Saturated Fat: 4g
- Cholesterol: 0mg
- Sodium: 400mg

Cheesy Ground Beef Quesadilla

Prep Time: 15 minutes
Cook Time: 15 minutes
Total Time: 30 minutes
Servings: 2 servings

Ingredients

- 1/2 pound lean ground beef
- 1 teaspoon olive oil

- 1/2 cup diced tomatoes
- 1/4 cup diced red onion
- 1/4 cup sliced black olives
- 1 teaspoon taco seasoning
- Salt and pepper to taste
- 2 whole wheat or low-carb tortillas
- 1 cup shredded low-fat cheddar or Monterey Jack cheese
- Cooking spray

Instructions

1. In a skillet, heat olive oil over medium heat. Using a spoon, break up the ground beef while it cooks until it turns brown.
2. Drain excess fat from the beef and add diced tomatoes, red onion, sliced black olives, taco seasoning, salt, and pepper. Cook for an additional 3-4 minutes.
3. Remove the beef mixture from the skillet and set aside.
4. Wipe the skillet with a paper towel and place it back on the heat.
5. Spray the skillet with cooking spray.
6. Lay one tortilla in the skillet and spread half of the shredded cheese evenly over it.
7. Spoon half of the beef mixture on top of the cheese.
8. Place the second tortilla on top.
9. Cook for about 2-3 minutes on each side or until the tortillas are golden brown and the cheese is melted.
10. Remove from the skillet, let it cool for a minute, then cut into wedges.
11. Repeat the process for the second quesadilla.

Nutritional Values (per serving)
- Calories: 400 kcal
- Protein: 25g
- Carbohydrates: 25g
- Dietary Fiber: 4g
- Sugars: 2g
- Fat: 20g
- Saturated Fat: 8g
- Cholesterol: 70mg
- Sodium: 500mg

Ground Beef & Broccoli Rice Bowl

Prep Time: 15 minutes
Cook Time: 20 minutes
Total Time: 35 minutes
Servings: 2 servings

Ingredients

- 1/2 pound lean ground beef
- 1 teaspoon olive oil
- 2 cups broccoli florets
- 1 cup cooked brown rice
- 2 tablespoons low-sodium soy sauce
- 1 tablespoon oyster sauce
- 1 teaspoon sesame oil
- 1 teaspoon grated ginger
- 2 cloves garlic, minced
- 1/4 teaspoon red pepper flakes (optional)
- Green onions for garnish (optional)
- Sesame seeds for garnish (optional)

Instructions

1. Heat the olive oil in a big skillet over medium heat. Using a spoon, break up the ground beef while it cooks until it turns brown.
2. Drain excess fat from the beef.
3. Add broccoli florets to the skillet and cook for 3-4 minutes until slightly tender.
4. In a small bowl, mix soy sauce, oyster sauce, sesame oil, grated ginger, minced garlic, and red pepper flakes if desired.
5. Add the cooked brown rice to the skillet, followed by the sauce mixture. Stir well to combine.
6. Cook for an additional 3-5 minutes until everything is heated through and well-coated with the sauce.
7. Remove from heat and garnish with green onions and sesame seeds if desired.
8. Serve immediately.

Nutritional Values (per serving)

- Calories: 400 kcal
- Protein: 25g
- Carbohydrates: 35g
- Dietary Fiber: 5g
- Sugars: 3g
- Fat: 18g
- Saturated Fat: 6g
- Cholesterol: 70mg
- Sodium: 600mg

Baked Furikake Salmon

Prep Time: 10 minutes
Marinating Time: 30 minutes
Cook Time: 15 minutes
Total Time: 55 minutes
Servings: 2 servings

Ingredients
- 2 salmon filets (about 6 ounces each)
- 2 tablespoons low-sodium soy sauce
- 1 tablespoon mirin (sweet rice wine)
- 1 teaspoon sesame oil
- 2 teaspoons furikake seasoning
- 1 teaspoon grated ginger
- 1 teaspoon minced garlic
- 1 tablespoon chopped green onions (for garnish, optional)
- Lemon wedges (for serving)

Instructions
1. Preheat the oven to 400°F (200°C).
2. In a small bowl, mix soy sauce, mirin, sesame oil, furikake seasoning, grated ginger, and minced garlic.
3. Pour the marinade over the salmon fillets in a shallow dish. Allow to marinate for at least 30 minutes in the refrigerator.
4. Line a baking sheet with parchment paper and place the marinated salmon fillets on it.
5. Bake for 12-15 minutes or until the salmon flakes easily with a fork.
6. If desired, garnish with chopped green onions.
7. Serve with lemon wedges.

Nutritional Values (per serving)
- Calories: 300 kcal
- Protein: 30g
- Carbohydrates: 5g
- Dietary Fiber: 1g
- Sugars: 2g
- Fat: 18g
- Saturated Fat: 3g
- Cholesterol: 80mg
- Sodium: 500mg

Air Fryer Mahi Mahi

Prep Time: 10 minutes
Marinating Time: 20 minutes
Cook Time: 12 minutes
Total Time: 42 minutes
Servings: 2 servings

Ingredients
- 2 Mahi Mahi filets (6 oz each)
- 1 tablespoon olive oil
- 1 tablespoon lemon juice
- 1 teaspoon dried herbs (such as thyme, rosemary, or oregano)
- 1/2 teaspoon garlic powder
- Salt and pepper to taste
- Lemon wedges (for serving)

Instructions
1. In a bowl, mix olive oil, lemon juice, dried herbs, garlic powder, salt, and pepper.
2. Place the Mahi Mahi fillets in a shallow dish and pour the marinade over them. Allow to marinate for at least 20 minutes in the refrigerator.
3. Preheat the air fryer to 375°F (190°C).
4. Place the marinated Mahi Mahi fillets in the air fryer basket.
5. Cook for 10-12 minutes, flipping halfway through, or until the fish is opaque and flakes easily with a fork.
6. Serve with lemon wedges.

Nutritional Values (per serving)
- Calories: 250 kcal
- Protein: 35g
- Carbohydrates: 2g
- Dietary Fiber: 0g
- Sugars: 0g
- Fat: 11g
- Saturated Fat: 2g
- Cholesterol: 120mg
- Sodium: 200mg

Baked Mediterranean Fish

Prep Time: 15 minutes
Marinating Time: 30 minutes
Cook Time: 20 minutes
Total Time: 1 hour 5 minutes

Servings: 2 servings

Ingredients
- 2 white fish filets (such as cod or tilapia), about 6 ounces each
- 2 tablespoons olive oil
- 1 tablespoon lemon juice
- 1 teaspoon dried oregano
- 1 teaspoon dried thyme
- 1 teaspoon minced garlic
- Salt and pepper to taste
- 1/2 cup cherry tomatoes, halved
- 1/4 cup pitted and sliced Kalamata olives
- 1/4 cup crumbled feta cheese
- Fresh parsley for garnish

Instructions
1. Preheat the oven to 375°F (190°C).
2. In a bowl, mix olive oil, lemon juice, dried oregano, dried thyme, minced garlic, salt, and pepper.
3. Place the fish filets in a shallow dish and pour the marinade over them. Allow to marinate for at least 30 minutes in the refrigerator.
4. Line a baking sheet with parchment paper and place the marinated fish fillets on it.
5. Scatter halved cherry tomatoes and sliced Kalamata olives around the fish.
6. Bake for 18-20 minutes or until the fish is cooked through and flakes easily with a fork.
7. Sprinkle crumbled feta cheese over the fish and bake for an additional 2 minutes or until the cheese is slightly melted.
8. Garnish with fresh parsley before serving.

Nutritional Values (per serving)
- Calories: 300 kcal
- Protein: 30g
- Carbohydrates: 5g
- Dietary Fiber: 2g
- Sugars: 2g
- Fat: 18g
- Saturated Fat: 4g
- Cholesterol: 70mg
- Sodium: 500mg

Baked Salmon with Dill Sauce

Prep Time: 10 minutes
Marinating Time: 30 minutes
Cook Time: 15 minutes
Total Time: 55 minutes
Servings: 2 servings

Ingredients

For Baked Salmon:
- 2 salmon filets (about 6 ounces each)
- 1 tablespoon olive oil
- 1 tablespoon lemon juice
- 1 teaspoon dried dill
- 1 teaspoon minced garlic
- Salt and pepper to taste
- Lemon slices for garnish

For Dill Sauce:
- 1/2 cup plain Greek yogurt
- 1 tablespoon chopped fresh dill
- 1 teaspoon Dijon mustard
- 1 teaspoon lemon juice
- Salt and pepper to taste

Instructions

1. Preheat the oven to 400°F (200°C).
2. In a bowl, mix olive oil, lemon juice, dried dill, minced garlic, salt, and pepper.
3. Pour the marinade over the salmon filets in a shallow dish. Allow to marinate for at least 30 minutes in the refrigerator.
4. Line a baking sheet with parchment paper and place the marinated salmon fillets on it. Serve each filet with a lemon slice.
5. Bake for 12-15 minutes or until the salmon is cooked through and flakes easily with a fork.
6. While the salmon is baking, prepare the dill sauce by mixing Greek yogurt, chopped fresh dill, Dijon mustard, lemon juice, salt, and pepper in a bowl.
7. Serve the baked salmon with a dollop of dill sauce.

Nutritional Values (per serving)

- Calories: 350 kcal
- Protein: 30g
- Carbohydrates: 5g
- Dietary Fiber: 1g
- Sugars: 3g
- Fat: 22g
- Saturated Fat: 4g
- Sodium: 200mg

Shrimp Quesadilla Recipe

Prep Time: 15 minutes
Cook Time: 10 minutes
Total Time: 25 minutes
Servings: 2 servings

Ingredients
- 1/2 pound medium shrimp, peeled and deveined
- 1 teaspoon olive oil
- 1 teaspoon chili powder
- 1/2 teaspoon ground cumin
- Salt and pepper to taste
- 2 whole wheat or low-carb tortillas
- 1/2 cup shredded low-fat Monterey Jack cheese
- 1/4 cup diced tomatoes
- 1/4 cup diced red onion
- 1/4 cup chopped fresh cilantro
- 1 tablespoon lime juice
- Cooking spray

Instructions
1. In a bowl, toss shrimp with olive oil, chili powder, ground cumin, salt, and pepper.
2. Heat a skillet over medium-high heat. Add the seasoned shrimp and cook for 2-3 minutes per side or until they are opaque and cooked through. Set aside once removed from the skillet.
3. Wipe the skillet with a paper towel and place it back on the heat.
4. Spray the skillet with cooking spray.
5. Lay one tortilla in the skillet and spread half of the shredded cheese evenly over it.
6. Arrange half of the cooked shrimp, diced tomatoes, diced red onion, and chopped cilantro on top.
7. Place the second tortilla on top.
8. Cook for about 2-3 minutes on each side or until the tortillas are golden brown, and the cheese is melted.
9. Remove from the skillet, let it cool for a minute, then cut into wedges.
10. Repeat the process for the second quesadilla.

Nutritional Values (per serving)
- Calories: 350 kcal
- Protein: 30g
- Carbohydrates: 25g
- Dietary Fiber: 5g
- Sugars: 3g
- Fat: 15g
- Saturated Fat: 5g
- Sodium: 500mg

Napa Cabbage Slaw

Prep Time: 15 minutes
Total Time: 15 minutes
Servings: 4 servings

Ingredients
- 4 cups thinly sliced Napa cabbage
- 1 cup shredded carrots
- 1/2 cup thinly sliced red bell pepper
- 1/4 cup chopped green onions
- 1/4 cup chopped fresh cilantro
- 2 tablespoons sesame oil
- 2 tablespoons rice vinegar
- 1 tablespoon low-sodium soy sauce
- 1 teaspoon grated ginger
- Sesame seeds for garnish (optional)

Instructions
1. In a large bowl, combine Napa cabbage, shredded carrots, sliced red bell pepper, chopped green onions, and chopped fresh cilantro.
2. In a small bowl, whisk together sesame oil, rice vinegar, low-sodium soy sauce, and grated ginger.
3. Toss the cabbage mixture with the dressing until evenly coated.
4. Let the slaw sit for a few minutes to allow the flavors to meld.
5. Garnish with sesame seeds if desired.
6. Serve immediately.

Nutritional Values (per serving)
- Calories: 80 kcal
- Protein: 2g
- Carbohydrates: 8g
- Dietary Fiber: 3g
- Sugars: 4g
- Fat: 5g
- Saturated Fat: 1g
- Cholesterol: 0mg
- Sodium: 210mg

Ground Pork Stir Fry with Peanut Sauce

Prep Time: 15 minutes
Cook Time: 15 minutes
Total Time: 30 minutes
Servings: 2 servings

Ingredients
For Stir Fry:
- 1/2 pound lean ground pork
- 1 tablespoon vegetable oil
- 2 cups broccoli florets
- 1 bell pepper, thinly sliced
- 1 carrot, julienned
- 2 cloves garlic, minced
- 1 tablespoon grated ginger
- Sesame seeds for garnish (optional)
- Chopped green onions for garnish (optional)

For Peanut Sauce:
- 2 tablespoons natural peanut butter (unsweetened)
- 2 tablespoons low-sodium soy sauce
- 1 tablespoon rice vinegar
- 1 tablespoon sesame oil
- 1 tsp honey (or sugar alternative)
- 1/2 teaspoon chili flakes (optional)
- 2-3 tablespoons water (to achieve desired consistency)

Instructions
1. In a bowl, mix ground pork with minced garlic and grated ginger.
2. In a large skillet over medium-high heat, heat the vegetable oil. Add the seasoned ground pork and cook until browned, breaking it apart with a spoon.
3. Add broccoli, bell pepper, and julienned carrot to the skillet. Stir-fry the vegetables for 3-4 minutes, or until they are tender-crisp.
4. In a small bowl, whisk together peanut butter, soy sauce, rice vinegar, sesame oil, honey (or sugar substitute), and chili flakes if desired. Add water gradually until you achieve the desired sauce consistency.
5. Pour the peanut sauce over the stir fry and toss until everything is well coated.
6. Cook for an additional 2-3 minutes until heated through.
7. Garnish with sesame seeds and chopped green onions if desired.
8. Serve immediately.

Nutritional Values (per serving)
- Calories: 400 kcal

- Protein: 25g
- Carbohydrates: 15g
- Dietary Fiber: 4g
- Sugars: 5g
- Fat: 28g
- Saturated Fat: 7g
- Cholesterol: 60mg
- Sodium: 600mg

Spaghetti Squash Turkey Parmesan

Prep Time: 15 minutes
Cook Time: 45 minutes
Total Time: 1 hour
Servings: 2 servings

Ingredients
- 1 medium spaghetti squash, peeled and halved
- 1 tablespoon olive oil
- Salt and pepper to taste
- 1/2 pound ground turkey
- 1 clove garlic, minced
- 1 cup sugar-free marinara sauce
- 1 teaspoon dried oregano
- 1 teaspoon dried basil
- 1/2 cup shredded mozzarella cheese
- 2 tablespoons grated Parmesan cheese
- Fresh basil for garnish (optional)

Instructions
1. Preheat the oven to 400°F (200°C).
2. Brush the cut sides of the spaghetti squash with olive oil and season with salt and pepper.
3. Place the squash on a baking pan, cut side down. Roast the squash for 40-45 minutes, or until soft.
4. While the squash is roasting, heat a skillet over medium heat. Add ground turkey and cook until the ground turkey is browned, breaking it up with a spoon.
5. Add minced garlic to the turkey and cook for an additional minute.
6. Stir in sugar-free marinara sauce, dried oregano, and dried basil. Simmer for 5-7 minutes.
7. Once the spaghetti squash is done, use a fork to scrape the strands into a bowl.
8. In an ovenproof dish, layer half of the spaghetti squash, followed by half of the turkey marinara mixture. Repeat with the remaining squash and turkey mixture.
9. Top with shredded mozzarella and grated Parmesan cheese.

10. Broil for 2-3 minutes or until the cheese is melted and bubbly.
11. Garnish with fresh basil if desired.
12. Serve immediately.

Nutritional Values (per serving)
- Calories: 350 kcal
- Protein: 25g
- Carbohydrates: 20g
- Dietary Fiber: 5g
- Sugars: 8g
- Fat: 18g
- Saturated Fat: 6g
- Cholesterol: 60mg
- Sodium: 600mg

In-N-Out Style Turkey Burger

Prep Time: 15 minutes
Cook Time: 10 minutes
Total Time: 25 minutes
Servings: 2 servings

Ingredients
For Turkey Patties:
- 1/2 pound ground turkey
- 1/4 teaspoon garlic powder
- 1/4 teaspoon onion powder
- Salt and pepper to taste

For Burger Assembly:
- 2 whole wheat or lettuce wrap buns
- 2 tablespoons sugar-free ketchup
- 2 tablespoons mustard
- 2 slices low-fat Swiss cheese
- Iceberg lettuce leaves
- Tomato slices
- Red onion slices
- Dill pickles

Instructions
1. In a bowl, mix ground turkey with garlic powder, onion powder, salt, and pepper. Form into two patties.
2. Heat a skillet or grill pan over medium-high heat. Cook the turkey patties for about 5 minutes per side or until fully cooked.

3. In the last minute of cooking, place a slice of low-fat Swiss cheese on each patty and cover to melt.
4. While the patties are cooking, assemble your lettuce wrap buns and prepare the toppings.
5. Spread sugar-free ketchup and mustard on the buns or lettuce leaves.
6. Place the cooked turkey patties with melted cheese on the prepared buns or lettuce wraps.
7. Top with iceberg lettuce, tomato slices, red onion slices, and dill pickles.
8. Secure the burger with a toothpick if needed.
9. Serve immediately.

Nutritional Values (per serving)
- Calories: 300 kcal
- Protein: 25g
- Carbohydrates: 15g
- Dietary Fiber: 3g
- Sugars: 2g
- Fat: 15g
- Saturated Fat: 5g
- Cholesterol: 70mg
- Sodium: 500mg

Grilled Lemon Garlic Chicken

Prep Time: 10 minutes
Marinating Time: 30 minutes
Cook Time: 15 minutes
Total Time: 55 minutes
Servings: 2 servings

Ingredients
- 2 boneless, skinless chicken breasts
- 2 tablespoons olive oil
- Zest of 1 lemon
- Juice of 1 lemon
- 3 cloves garlic, minced
- 1 teaspoon dried oregano
- Salt and pepper to taste
- Fresh parsley for garnish (optional)
- Lemon wedges for serving

Instructions

1. In a bowl, whisk together olive oil, lemon zest, lemon juice, minced garlic, dried oregano, salt, and pepper.
2. Place the chicken breasts in a shallow dish and pour the marinade over them. Ensure the chicken is well coated. Marinate for at least 30 minutes in the refrigerator.
3. Preheat the grill to medium-high heat.
4. Remove the chicken from the marinade and let excess marinade drip off.
5. Grill the chicken for about 6-8 minutes per side or until fully cooked and grill marks appear.
6. Baste the chicken with any remaining marinade during grilling.
7. Let the chicken rest for a few minutes before slicing.
8. Garnish with fresh parsley if desired and serve with lemon wedges.

Nutritional Values (per serving)

- Calories: 250 kcal
- Protein: 30g
- Carbohydrates: 2g
- Dietary Fiber: 0g
- Sugars: 0g
- Fat: 13g
- Saturated Fat: 2g
- Cholesterol: 80mg
- Sodium: 100mg

Turkey Burger Sliders

Prep Time: 15 minutes
Cook Time: 10 minutes
Total Time: 25 minutes
Servings: 2 servings (4 sliders)

Ingredients
For Turkey Patties:
- 1/2 pound ground turkey
- 1/4 teaspoon garlic powder
- 1/4 teaspoon onion powder
- Salt and pepper to taste

For Slider Assembly:
- 4 whole wheat or lettuce wrap slider buns
- 2 tablespoons sugar-free ketchup
- 2 tablespoons mustard
- 4 small low-fat Swiss cheese slices
- Iceberg lettuce leaves

- Tomato slices
- Red onion slices
- Dill pickles

Instructions

1. In a bowl, mix ground turkey with garlic powder, onion powder, salt, and pepper. Form into four small patties.
2. Heat a skillet or grill pan over medium-high heat. Cook the turkey patties for about 3-4 minutes per side or until fully cooked.
3. In the last minute of cooking, place a slice of low-fat Swiss cheese on each patty and cover to melt.
4. While the patties are cooking, assemble your slider buns and prepare the toppings.
5. Spread sugar-free ketchup and mustard on the buns or lettuce leaves.
6. Place the cooked turkey patties with melted cheese on the prepared buns or lettuce wraps.
7. Top with iceberg lettuce, tomato slices, red onion slices, and dill pickles.
8. Secure the sliders with toothpicks if needed.
9. Serve immediately.

Nutritional Values (per serving - 2 sliders)

- Calories: 300 kcal
- Protein: 25g
- Carbohydrates: 15g
- Dietary Fiber: 3g
- Sugars: 2g
- Fat: 15g
- Saturated Fat: 5g
- Cholesterol: 70mg
- Sodium: 500mg

Crockpot Chicken & Salsa

Prep Time: 10 minutes
Cook Time: 4-6 hours on low
Total Time: 4-6 hours, 10 minutes
Servings: 4 servings

Ingredients

- 4 boneless, skinless chicken breasts
- 2 cups salsa (choose a sugar-free or low-sugar option)
- 1 teaspoon ground cumin
- 1 teaspoon chili powder
- 1/2 teaspoon garlic powder
- Salt and pepper to taste

- Fresh cilantro for garnish (optional)

Instructions
1. Place the chicken breasts in the slow cooker.
2. In a bowl, mix salsa, ground cumin, chili powder, garlic powder, salt, and pepper.
3. Pour the salsa mixture over the chicken, ensuring it's well coated.
4. Cover and cook on low for 4-6 hours or until the chicken is cooked through and easily shredded.
5. Once cooked, shred the chicken using two forks and mix it with the salsa mixture.
6. Serve over cauliflower rice, in lettuce wraps, or with your preferred low-carb sides.
7. Garnish with fresh cilantro if desired.

Nutritional Values (per serving)
- Calories: 200 kcal
- Protein: 25g
- Carbohydrates: 8g
- Dietary Fiber: 2g
- Sugars: 4g
- Fat: 7g
- Saturated Fat: 1.5g
- Cholesterol: 70mg
- Sodium: 600mg

CHAPTER FOUR: SNACKS AND DESSERT

Mixed Nut & Popcorn

Ingredients

- 1 cup mixed nuts (almonds, walnuts, and pecans)
- 4 cups air-popped popcorn
- 1 tablespoon olive oil
- 1 teaspoon smoked paprika
- 1/2 teaspoon garlic powder
- 1/2 teaspoon onion powder
- 1/4 teaspoon cayenne pepper (optional)
- Salt to taste

Instructions

1. In a large mixing bowl, combine mixed nuts.
2. In a small bowl, mix olive oil, smoked paprika, garlic powder, onion powder, cayenne pepper (if using), and salt.
3. Drizzle the spice mixture over the nuts and toss until evenly coated.
4. Preheat your oven to 350°F (175°C).
5. Spread the seasoned nuts on a baking sheet and roast for about 10-12 minutes or until they are toasted and fragrant. Keep an eye on them to avoid burning.
6. While the nuts are roasting, air-pop the popcorn.
7. Once the nuts are done, let them cool slightly.
8. In a large bowl, mix the roasted nuts with the air-popped popcorn.
9. Allow the snack to cool completely before serving.

Nutritional Values (per serving - 1 cup)
- Calories: 250 kcal
- Protein: 8g
- Carbohydrates: 20g
- Dietary Fiber: 5g
- Sugars: 0g
- Fat: 18g
- Saturated Fat: 2g
- Cholesterol: 0mg
- Sodium: 100mg

Apple Slices

Ingredients
- 2 medium-sized apples (choose a variety with lower sugar content)
- 1 tablespoon unsweetened almond or peanut butter
- 1 teaspoon cinnamon
- 1 tablespoon chopped nuts (e.g., almonds, walnuts) for added crunch (optional)
- Fresh lemon juice (to prevent browning)

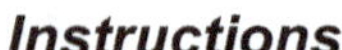

Instructions
1. Wash and slice the apples into thin wedges.
2. Place the apple slices in a bowl and drizzle fresh lemon juice over them to prevent browning.
3. In a small dish, warm the almond or peanut butter for a few seconds in the microwave.
4. Drizzle the warm nut butter over the apple slices.
5. Sprinkle cinnamon evenly over the apple slices.
6. Optionally, add chopped nuts for extra crunch.
7. Toss the apple slices gently until they are well coated with the nut butter and cinnamon.
8. Serve immediately.

Nutritional Values (per serving)
- Calories: 150 kcal
- Protein: 2g
- Carbohydrates: 25g
- Dietary Fiber: 5g
- Sugars: 18g
- Fat: 6g
- Saturated Fat: 0.5g
- Cholesterol: 0mg
- Sodium: 0mg

Deviled Eggs & Kiwi

Ingredients
For Deviled Eggs:
- 4 hard-boiled eggs, peeled
- 2 tablespoons Greek yogurt
- 1 teaspoon Dijon mustard
- 1 teaspoon fresh lemon juice
- Salt and pepper to taste
- Paprika for garnish
For Kiwi:
- 2 ripe kiwis, peeled and sliced

Instructions
1. Cut the hard-boiled eggs in half lengthwise.
2. Remove the yolks with care and place them in a basin.
3. Mash the yolks with a fork and mix in Greek yogurt, Dijon mustard, fresh lemon juice, salt, and pepper until smooth.
4. Spoon or pipe the yolk mixture back into the egg white halves.
5. Sprinkle with paprika for garnish.
6. Peel and cut the kiwis into rounds.
7. Arrange the deviled eggs and kiwi slices on a plate.
8. Serve immediately.

Nutritional Values (per serving)
- Calories: 180 kcal
- Protein: 10g
- Carbohydrates: 14g
- Dietary Fiber: 3g
- Sugars: 7g
- Fat: 10g
- Saturated Fat: 3g
- Cholesterol: 380mg
- Sodium: 150mg

Coconut Macaroons

Prep Time: 15 minutes
Cook Time: 20 minutes
Total Time: 35 minutes
Servings: 12 macaroons

Ingredients
- 3 cups shredded unsweetened coconut
- 1/2 cup almond flour
- 1/2 cup erythritol or sweetener of choice
- 1/4 teaspoon salt
- 3 egg whites
- 1 teaspoon vanilla extract

Instructions
1. Preheat your oven to 325°F (163°C) and line a baking sheet with parchment paper.
2. In a large bowl, combine shredded coconut, almond flour, sweetener, and salt.
3. In a separate dish, beat the egg whites until stiff peaks form.
4. Gently fold the whipped egg whites into the coconut mixture, and add vanilla extract.
5. Using a cookie scoop or your hands, form the mixture into small mounds and place them on the prepared baking sheet.
6. Bake for 15-20 minutes, or until golden brown around the edges.
7. Allow the macaroons to cool on the baking sheet before transferring to a wire rack.

Nutritional Values (per macaroon)
- Calories: 120
- Total Fat: 10g
- Saturated Fat: 9g
- Cholesterol: 0mg
- Sodium: 50mg
- Total Carbohydrates: 5g
- Dietary Fiber: 3g
- Sugars: 1g
- Protein: 2g

Banana Oat Cookies

Prep Time: 10 minutes
Cook Time: 15 minutes
Total Time: 25 minutes
Servings: 15 cookies

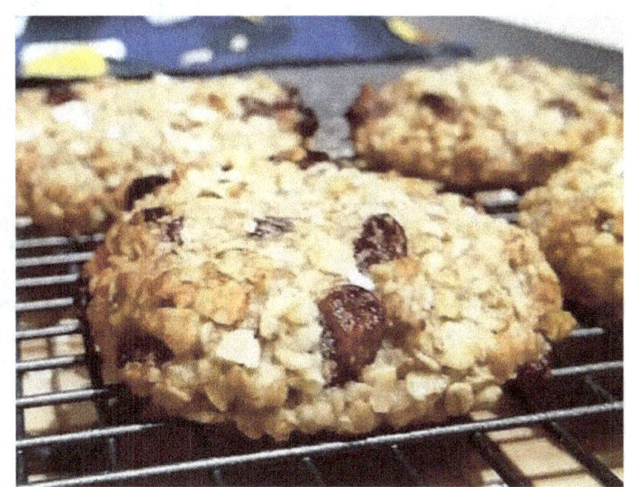

Ingredients
- 2 ripe bananas, mashed
- 1 1/2 cups rolled oats
- 1/2 cup almond flour
- 1/4 cup coconut oil, melted
- 1/4 cup honey or maple syrup
- 1/2 teaspoon vanilla extract
- 1/2 teaspoon cinnamon
- 1/4 teaspoon salt

Instructions
1. Preheat your oven to 350°F (177°C) and line a baking sheet with parchment paper.
2. In a large bowl, combine mashed bananas, rolled oats, almond flour, melted coconut oil, honey (or maple syrup), vanilla extract, cinnamon, and salt.
3. Mix until well combined, ensuring the oats are evenly coated.
4. Using a spoon, drop cookie dough onto the prepared baking sheet, shaping each into a cookie.
5. Bake for 12-15 minutes or until the edges turn golden brown.
6. Allow the cookies to cool on the baking sheet for a few minutes before transferring them to a wire rack.

Nutritional Values (per cookie)
- Calories: 90
- Total Fat: 4g
- Saturated Fat: 2g
- Cholesterol: 0mg
- Sodium: 30mg
- Total Carbohydrates: 13g
- Dietary Fiber: 2g
- Sugars: 5g
- Protein: 2g

Sugar-free Chocolate Truffles

Prep Time: 20 minutes
Chill Time: 2 hours
Total Time: 2 hours 20 minutes
Servings: 20 truffles

Ingredients
- 1 cup dark chocolate chips (sugar-free)
- 1/2 cup coconut cream
- 2 tablespoons unsweetened cocoa powder
- 1 teaspoon vanilla extract
- A pinch of salt
- Coating options: unsweetened cocoa powder, chopped nuts, or shredded coconut

Instructions
1. In a heatproof bowl, melt the sugar-free dark chocolate chips using a double boiler or microwave in short intervals, stirring until smooth.
2. Heat the coconut cream until warm, not boiling, and then add it to the melted chocolate. Mix well.
3. Stir in the unsweetened cocoa powder, vanilla extract, and a pinch of salt. Combine until the mixture is smooth and glossy.
4. Cover the bowl and refrigerate the chocolate mixture for at least 2 hours or until it's firm enough to handle.
5. Once chilled, scoop out small portions and roll them into truffle-sized balls.
6. Roll each truffle in your preferred coating: unsweetened cocoa powder, chopped nuts, or shredded coconut.
7. Place the coated truffles on a plate and refrigerate for an additional 15-20 minutes.

Nutritional Values (per truffle)
- Calories: 60
- Total Fat: 5g
- Saturated Fat: 3g
- Cholesterol: 0mg
- Sodium: 5mg
- Total Carbohydrates: 5g
- Dietary Fiber: 2g
- Sugars: 0g
- Protein: 1g

Baked Pears

Prep Time: 10 minutes
Bake Time: 25 minutes
Total Time: 35 minutes
Servings: 4

Ingredients
- 4 ripe but firm pears, halved and cored
- 1 tablespoon melted coconut oil
- 2 tablespoons honey or maple syrup
- 1 teaspoon cinnamon
- 1/4 cup chopped walnuts or almonds
(optional)

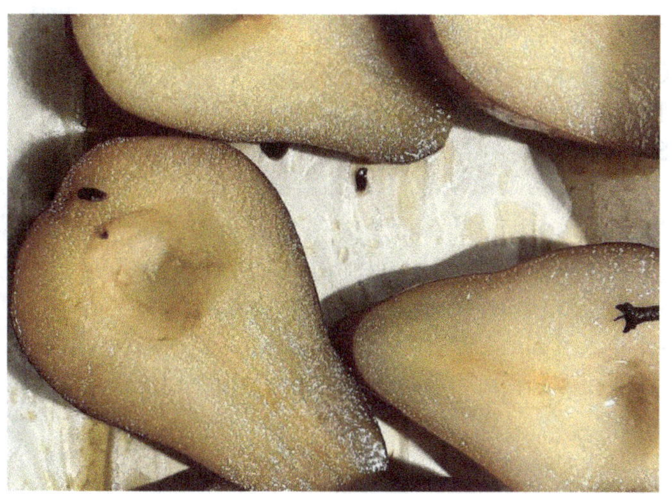

Instructions
1. Preheat the oven to 375°F (190°C) and prepare a baking dish with parchment paper.
2. Arrange the pear halves cut side up in the baking dish.
3. In a small bowl, mix together melted coconut oil, honey (or maple syrup), and cinnamon.
4. Brush the mixture over each pear half, ensuring they are well coated.
5. If desired, sprinkle chopped nuts over the top of each pear.
6. Bake in the preheated oven for 25 minutes or until the pears are tender and golden.
7. Remove from the oven and set aside to cool before serving.

Nutritional Values (per serving)
- Calories: 120
- Total Fat: 4g
- Saturated Fat: 2.5g
- Cholesterol: 0mg
- Sodium: 0mg
- Total Carbohydrates: 24g
- Dietary Fiber: 4g
- Sugars: 16g
- Protein: 1g

Chocolate Avocado Mousse

Prep Time: 10 minutes
Chill Time: 1 hour
Total Time: 1 hour 10 minutes
Servings: 4

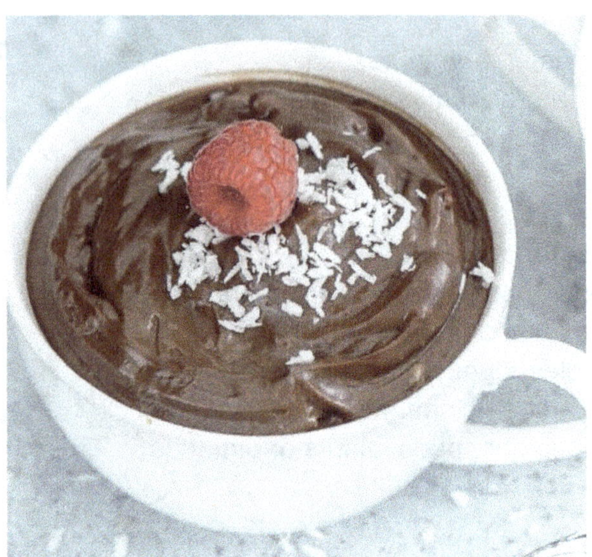

Ingredients
- 2 ripe avocados, peeled and pitted
- 1/4 cup unsweetened cocoa powder
- 1/4 cup almond milk (unsweetened)
- 1/4 cup sugar-free sweetener (adjust to taste)
- 1 teaspoon vanilla extract
- A pinch of salt
- Optional toppings: berries, mint leaves, or chopped nuts

Instructions
1. In a blender or food processor, combine the ripe avocados, cocoa powder, almond milk, sugar-free sweetener, vanilla extract, and a pinch of salt.
2. Blend until smooth and creamy.
3. Taste and adjust the sweetness if needed.
4. Divide the chocolate avocado mousse into serving glasses or bowls.
5. Refrigerate the mousse for at least 1 hour to allow it to firm.
6. Before serving, add optional toppings such as berries, mint leaves, or chopped nuts.

Nutritional Values (per serving)
- Calories: 150
- Total Fat: 12g
- Saturated Fat: 2g
- Cholesterol: 0mg
- Sodium: 10mg
- Total Carbohydrates: 11g
- Dietary Fiber: 7g
- Sugars: 1g
- Protein: 3g

Kale Chips

Prep Time: 10 minutes
Bake Time: 15 minutes
Total Time: 25 minutes
Servings: 4

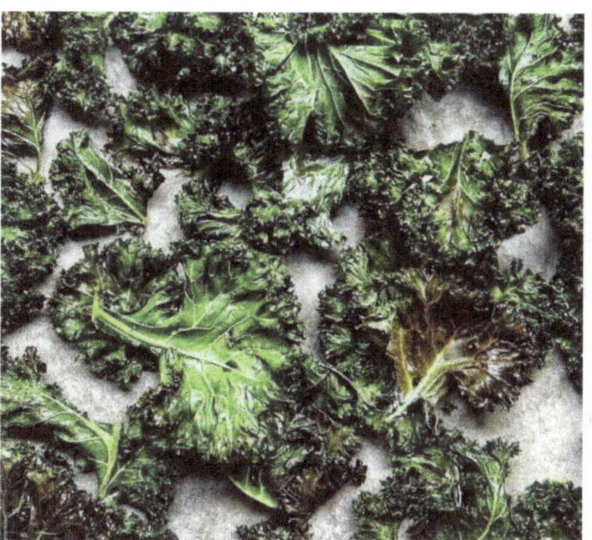

Ingredients
- 1 bunch kale, stems removed and leaves ripped into bite-sized pieces
- 1 tablespoon olive oil
- 1/2 teaspoon garlic powder
- 1/2 teaspoon onion powder
- 1/4 teaspoon smoked paprika
- Salt and pepper to taste

Instructions
1. Preheat your oven to 350°F (177°C) and line a baking sheet with parchment paper.
2. In a large bowl, toss kale pieces with olive oil, ensuring each leaf is lightly coated.
3. Sprinkle garlic powder, onion powder, smoked paprika, salt, and pepper over the kale. Toss one more to spread the ingredients evenly.
4. Spread the seasoned kale in a single layer on the prepared baking sheet.
5. Bake in the preheated oven for 12-15 minutes or until the edges are crisp and slightly golden.
6. Remove from the oven and let the kale chips cool on the baking sheet for a few minutes before transferring them to a serving bowl.

Nutritional Values (per serving)
- Calories: 60
- Total Fat: 4g
- Saturated Fat: 0.5g
- Cholesterol: 0mg
- Sodium: 25mg
- Total Carbohydrates: 5g
- Dietary Fiber: 1g
- Sugars: 0g
- Protein: 2g

Peanut Butter Fudge

Prep Time: 10 minutes
Chill Time: 2 hours
Total Time: 2 hours 10 minutes
Servings: 16 squares

Ingredients

- 1 cup natural peanut butter
- 1/2 cup coconut oil, melted
- 1/4 cup sugar-free sweetener (adjust to taste)
- 1 teaspoon vanilla extract
- A pinch of salt

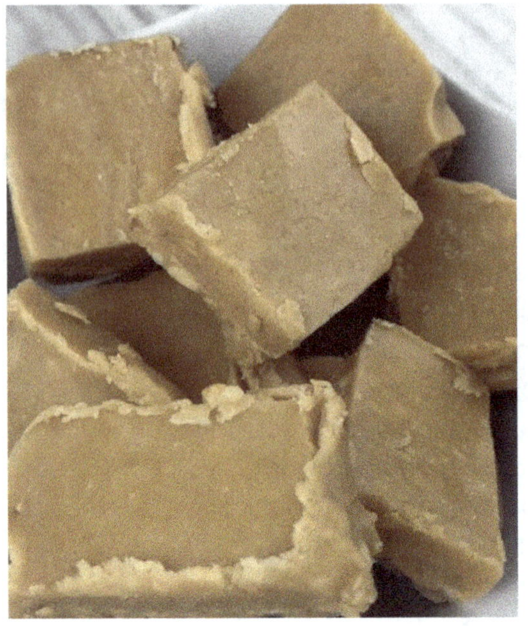

Instructions

1. Line a square baking dish with parchment paper, providing an overhang on all sides to allow for easy removal afterward.
2. In a microwave-safe bowl, melt the coconut oil.
3. Stir in the natural peanut butter, sugar-free sweetener, vanilla extract, and a pinch of salt until well combined.
4. Pour the mixture into the prepared baking dish, spreading it evenly.
5. Refrigerate for at least 2 hours or until the fudge is set.
6. Once set, use the parchment paper overhang to lift the fudge from the dish.
7. Cut into 16 squares and enjoy!

Nutritional Values (per square)

- Calories: 120
- Total Fat: 11g
- Saturated Fat: 6g
- Cholesterol: 0mg
- Sodium: 30mg
- Total Carbohydrates: 3g
- Dietary Fiber: 1g
- Sugars: 1g
- Protein: 3g

Pumpkin Scones

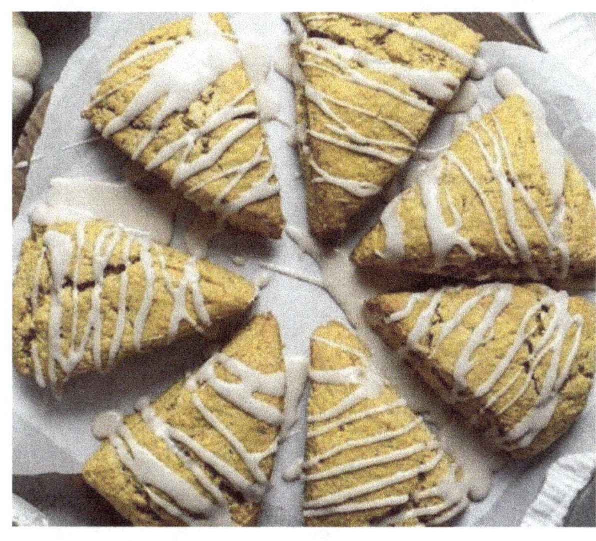

Prep Time: 15 minutes
Bake Time: 18 minutes
Total Time: 33 minutes
Servings: 8 scones

Ingredients
- 2 cups almond flour
- 1/4 cup coconut flour
- 1/4 cup sugar-free sweetener (adjust to taste)
- 1 teaspoon baking powder
- 1/2 teaspoon baking soda
- 1/2 teaspoon cinnamon
- 1/4 teaspoon nutmeg
- 1/4 teaspoon salt
- 1/2 cup pumpkin puree
- 1/4 cup coconut oil, melted
- 1 large egg
- 1 teaspoon vanilla extract
- Optional glaze: mix of powdered sugar substitute and almond milk

Instructions
1. Preheat your oven to 350°F (177°C) and line a baking sheet with parchment paper.
2. In a large bowl, whisk together almond flour, coconut flour, sugar-free sweetener, baking powder, baking soda, cinnamon, nutmeg, and salt.
3. In a separate bowl, combine pumpkin puree, melted coconut oil, egg, and vanilla extract.
4. Mix the wet and dry ingredients together until a dough forms.
5. Transfer the dough to a lightly floured surface and shape it into a circle about 1 inch thick.
6. Cut the circle into 8 wedges and place them on the prepared baking sheet.
7. Bake for 18 minutes or until the scones are golden brown.
8. Allow the scones to cool on the baking sheet before drizzling with the optional glaze.

Nutritional Values (per scone)
- Calories: 220
- Total Fat: 19g
- Saturated Fat: 7g
- Cholesterol: 25mg
- Sodium: 180mg
- Total Carbohydrates: 8g
- Dietary Fiber: 4g
- Sugars: 1g
- Protein: 6g

Pumpkin Pie

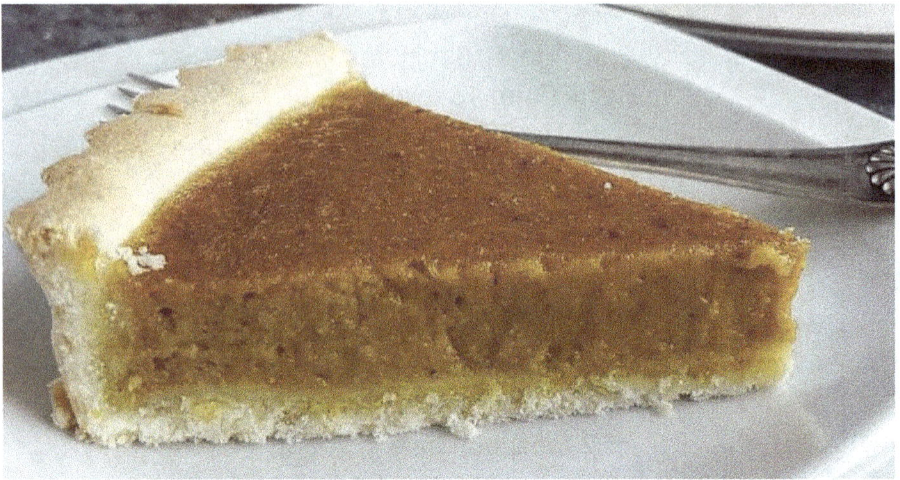

Prep Time: 20 minutes
Bake Time: 50 minutes
Cool Time: 2 hours
Total Time: 3 hours 10 minutes
Servings: 8 slices

Ingredients
- 1 1/2 cups canned pumpkin puree
- 1/2 cup coconut milk (full fat)
- 2 large eggs
- 1/2 cup sugar-free sweetener (adjust to taste)
- 1 teaspoon cinnamon
- 1/2 teaspoon ground ginger
- 1/4 teaspoon ground cloves
- 1/4 teaspoon nutmeg
- 1/4 teaspoon salt
- 1 pre-made almond flour pie crust (or your preferred low-carb crust)

Instructions
1. Preheat your oven to 350°F (177°C).
2. In a large bowl, whisk together pumpkin puree, coconut milk, eggs, sugar-free sweetener, cinnamon, ginger, cloves, nutmeg, and salt until well combined.
3. Pour the pumpkin mixture into the pre-made almond flour pie crust.
4. Bake in the preheated oven for 50 minutes or until the center is set.
5. Remove from the oven and let the pie cool completely on a wire rack.
6. Once cooled, refrigerate for at least 2 hours before slicing and serving.

Nutritional Values (per slice)
- Calories: 180
- Total Fat: 15g

- Saturated Fat: 6g
- Cholesterol: 45mg
- Sodium: 140mg
- Total Carbohydrates: 10g
- Dietary Fiber: 4g
- Sugars: 1g
- Protein: 4g

Lemon Cheesecake

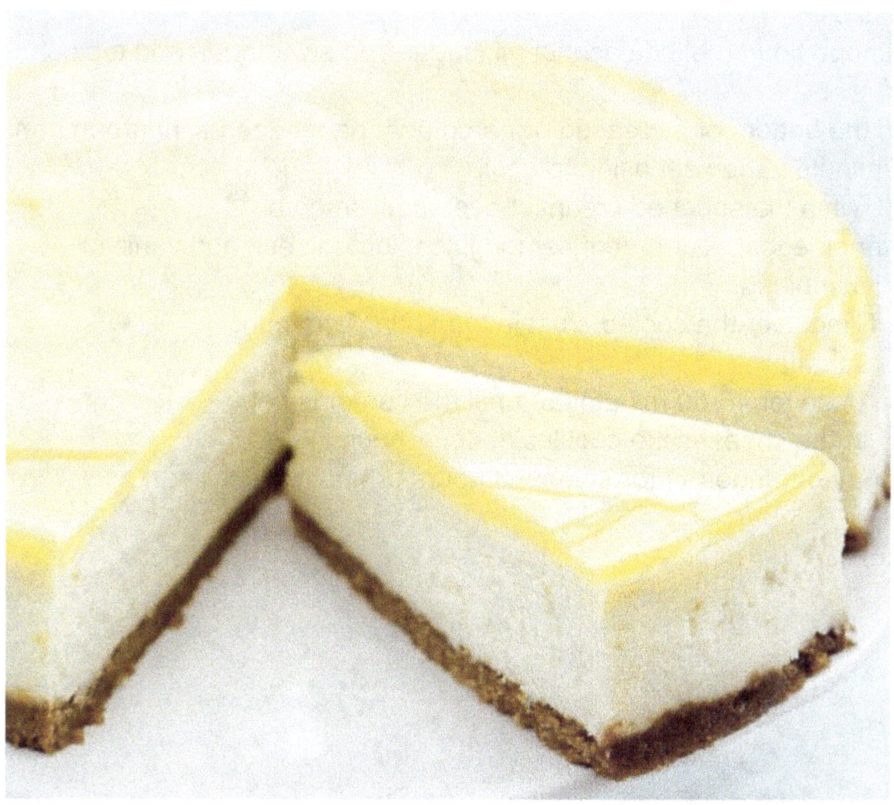

Prep Time: 20 minutes
Chill Time: 4 hours
Total Time: 4 hours 20 minutes
Servings: 10 slices

Ingredients
For the Crust
- 1 1/2 cups almond flour
- 1/4 cup coconut oil, melted
- 1/4 cup sugar-free sweetener (adjust to taste)
- A pinch of salt

For the Cheesecake Filling
- 16 oz cream cheese, softened
- 1 cup sugar-free sweetener (adjust to taste)
- 3 large eggs
- 1/2 cup sour cream
- 1/4 cup fresh lemon juice
- Zest of 1 lemon
- 1 teaspoon vanilla extract

Instructions

1. Preheat your oven to 325°F (163°C).
2. In a bowl, combine almond flour, melted coconut oil, sugar-free sweetener, and a pinch of salt.
3. Press the mixture into the bottom of a greased or parchment paper-lined springform pan.
4. Bake the crust for 10 minutes, then set aside to cool.
5. In a large mixing bowl, whip the softened cream cheese until smooth.
6. Add sugar-free sweetener, eggs, sour cream, lemon juice, lemon zest, and vanilla extract. Beat until well combined.
7. Pour the cheesecake filling over the cooled crust in the springform pan.
8. Smooth the top with a spatula.
9. Bake in the preheated oven for 45-50 minutes or until the center is set.
10. Turn off the oven and let the cheesecake cool inside for 1 hour.
11. Remove from the oven and refrigerate for at least 3 hours or until fully chilled.

Nutritional Values (per slice)
- Calories: 300
- Total Fat: 28g
- Saturated Fat: 15g
- Cholesterol: 110mg
- Sodium: 200mg
- Total Carbohydrates: 7g
- Dietary Fiber: 2g
- Sugars: 1g
- Protein: 7g

MEAL PLAN

Day 1:
- Breakfast: Greek Yogurt Parfait
- Lunch: Tuscan White Bean Soup
- Dinner: Chicken Stir Fry
- Snack: Mixed Nut & Popcorn

Day 2:
- Breakfast: Peanut Butter Overnight Oats
- Lunch: Chicken Cheese Quesadilla
- Dinner: Baked Furikake Salmon
- Snack: Apple Slices

Day 3:
- Breakfast: High Protein Pancakes
- Lunch: Ground Pork Stir Fry with Peanut Sauce
- Dinner: Spicy Sweet Potato Soup
- Snack: Deviled Eggs & Kiwi

Day 4:
- Breakfast: Chia Seed Pudding with Raspberries
- Lunch: Turkey Burger & Sweet Potato Fries
- Dinner: Baked Mediterranean Fish
- Snack: Coconut Macaroons

Day 5:
- Breakfast: Breakfast Burritos
- Lunch: Napa Cabbage Slaw
- Dinner: Grilled Lemon Garlic Chicken
- Snack: Banana Oat Cookies

Day 6:
- Breakfast: Tofu & Veggies Scramble
- Lunch: Spaghetti Squash Turkey Parmesan
- Dinner: Turkey Burger Sliders
- Snack: Sugar-free Chocolate Truffles

Day 7:
- Breakfast: Quinoa Porridge
- Lunch: In-N-Out Style Turkey Burger
- Dinner: Crockpot Chicken & Salsa
- Snack: Baked Pears

Day 8:
- Breakfast: Protein Smoothie
- Lunch: Quinoa Arugula Salad with Lemon Vinaigrette
- Dinner: Ground Beef & Broccoli Rice Bowl
- Snack: Kale Chips

Day 9:
- Breakfast: Egg Muffins
- Lunch: Rotisserie Chicken Salad
- Dinner: Air Fryer Mahi Mahi
- Snack: Peanut Butter Fudge

Day 10:
- Breakfast: Hard Boiled Eggs with Soldiers
- Lunch: Chicken Drumsticks, Zucchini Fries, & Brown Rice
- Dinner: Shrimp Quesadilla Recipe
- Snack: Pumpkin Scones

CONCLUSION

To sum up, "Quick and Easy Gestational Diabetes Meals" is a credible and invaluable tool for anyone navigating the difficulties associated with gestational diabetes. With an emphasis on ease of use, speed, and nutrition, this book offers more than simply recipes—it also serves as a guide for making wise nutritional decisions during this critical time.

As you turn the final pages, you will have a repertoire of tasty, well-balanced meals tailored to the particular nutritional requirements of people with gestational diabetes. The focus on speedy preparation guarantees that the demands of a busy lifestyle do not compromise the dedication to health.

Beyond the food, this book promotes understanding and self-determination. It provides useful advice on how to prepare meals that not only control blood sugar levels but also nourish the body and promote the health of the mother and unborn child. It demystifies the complexity of gestational diabetes.

By adopting the values presented in these pages, you set out on a path toward well-being and self-care. These recipes are more than just dinners; they're resilience tools that provide you the ability to deal with gestational diabetes problems in a graceful and fulfilling way.

I hope that the dishes included in these covers will satisfy your appetite and bring you a sense of empowerment and control over your health path. Here's to celebrating the happy expectation of a new life while simultaneously relishing the delight of nutritious, fast, and easy meals that satisfy the nutritional needs of gestational diabetes. May you take this book's insight and cooking inspiration with you, and may your pregnancy journey be fruitful and safe.

Thank you!